INTERN

CLEANSING

Revised
2nd Edition

· ·

RID

YOUR

BODY

OF

TOXINS

· ·

LINDA BERRY, D.C., C.C.N.

 THREE RIVERS PRESS · NEW YORK

Published by Three Rivers Press, New York, New York.
Member of the Crown Publishing Group, a division of Random House, Inc.
www.crownpublishing.com

THREE RIVERS PRESS and the Tugboat design are registered trademarks of Random House, Inc.

Originally published by Prima Publishing, Roseville, California, in 2001.

Warning—Disclaimer
This book is not intended to provide medical advice and is sold with the understanding that the publisher and the author are not liable for the misconception or misuse of information provided. The author and Random House, Inc., shall have neither liability nor responsibility to any person or entity with respect to any loss, damage, or injury caused or alleged to be caused directly or indirectly by the information contained in this book or the use of any products mentioned. Readers should not use any of the products discussed in this book without the advice of a medical professional. The statements in this book have not been evaluated by the Food and Drug Administration. This information is not intended to diagnose, treat, cure, or prevent any disease.

Printed in the United States of America

Library of Congress Cataloging-in-Publication Data
Berry, Linda.
    Internal cleansing : rid your body of toxins / Linda Berry.—2nd ed.
      p. cm.
    Includes bibliographical references and index.
    1. Toxicology—Popular works. 2. Health. I. Title.
RA1213.B47 2000
613—dc21   00-058886

ISBN 0-7615-2932-2

10 9 8 7 6
Second Edition

This book is dedicated to you, the reader, in acknowledgment of your pursuit of better health. As we recognize the need for self-improvement and take steps in that direction, we also improve the health of our families, our communities, and the planet on which we live. In so doing, we honor the force that gives us life. Congratulations on your efforts!

It is generally not the disease but ignorance or neglect of the remedy which undermines the quality of one's life.

— *Mark Percival, D.C., N.D.,*
founder of Health Coach Systems International, Inc.

CONTENTS

FOREWORD

Through my 28 years in medical practice and health care as well as my personal and professional experience in juice fasting and detoxification, I have come to believe that the cleansing/detoxification process is the missing link in Western nutrition and one of the keys to real healing. I have seen hundreds of patients over the years transform regular or persistent illness into health and greatly improved vitality.

When we embark upon a purification process, we instinctively take more time for ourselves and make our health a higher priority, whereby we are inspired to reevaluate our life, activities, habits, relationships, and more. We are then motivated to make new goals for our future. These goals usually involve making habit changes, such as letting go of daily abuses of sugar, caffeine, alcohol, nicotine, and junk foods. We also are inspired and guided to make decisions and take actions that we have sensed were important but about which we had procrastinated or made excuses. Now we feel clear and present enough to make these changes in our work and career, home, relationships, and health.

One of my favorite experiences in medical practice is when I see the many positive side effects of natural therapies, especially from the cleansing process. Some of these wonderful side effects include reducing symptoms, elevating energy and attitude, and looking and feeling younger. I also receive many letters from readers who follow the guidelines in my books and experience improved health and many other positive changes in their lives.

More specifically, some of the medical concerns that I believe are related to toxicity and which respond well to detoxification are allergies, arthritis, elevated cholesterol, high blood pressure, fatigue and sluggishness, backaches, body pains, and gastrointestinal disorders. In reality, most of the medical problems that take many years to develop and which we often label as chronic degenerative diseases respond well to cleansing therapies, as well as other natural therapies and lifestyle modifications.

Dr. Linda Berry offers us a fresh, clear voice in her simple, practical purification guidebook, *Internal Cleansing*. Dr. Berry first helps us to understand the many areas of potential stress in our lives and the problems that may occur; then she helps to orient us to the many things we can do, with lifestyle and natural therapies to help alleviate stress and clean and clear our bodies from the inside out. Linda also provides many practical references for us to pursue further knowledge and support from her many helpful guidelines.

I recommend this book highly as a useful guide to improving health and not just treating symptoms or disease. Since I believe that cleansing the body and mind is a process crucial to long-term health with vitality, and a key way to attain and maintain health for the 21st century, we must be aware of sources of toxicity that surround us so we can protect ourselves from them. *Internal Cleansing* by Dr. Linda Berry provides us with the beginning steps and long-range guidance by helping us to be informed and gives us the how-to's to reach for that next level of health and our optimal potential.

ELSON M. HAAS, M.D.

Dr. Elson M. Haas is the founder and medical director of the Preventive Medical Center of

Marin, an integrated health-care facility in San Rafael, California. He is also the author of seven popular health books, including the new *False Fat Diet* (Ballantine Publishing Group), *The Staying Healthy Shopper's Guide* (Celestial Arts), and *Vitamins for Dummies* (IDG Books).

ACKNOWLEDGMENTS

Many people have been instrumental in the formation of this book. First, I would like to thank the entire staff at Prima and Crown, both those known to me and those not known, for getting the good word out about achieving vibrant health through cleansing. And, not in order of importance, thank you also to Peter, Mark, Cheri, the Jeffs, Nick, Dr. Lukaczer, Chris, Gary, and Ritamarie for your assistance, encouragement, and/or resources. Thank you to all of my patients who have taught and inspired me with your quest for health. And finally, I would like to acknowledge the divine from which all of this emanates.

DO YOU NEED INTERNAL CLEANSING?

The power that made our body can heal our body. Each of us has within us the power to heal our pain and dysfunctions. In my years of practice as a doctor of chiropractic and fifteen years as a Health Coach (see "What Is Health Coach?" page xvi), I have come to understand life as a balance of forces. Your daily choices determine your stress load and your ability to heal. As you improve your lifestyle and minimize your negative reaction to stress, you increase your internal resilience and consequently improve your health and well-being.

Our bodies are the temples of our souls, and as such they deserve kind attention. Too often we neglect our health, placing our job, family, clients, and even our pets before ourselves. Instead of caring for ourselves and nourishing our body/mind/spirit, we often stuff ourselves full of harmful substances and influences that lead to blockage and congestion within our system. A safe, simple, and effective way to begin transforming negative, constipated energies is to cleanse your body so that it may serve rather than hinder your mind and soul, and cease interfering with your ability to perform your life's work.

Some people are motivated by pain; others are motivated by pleasure. What motivates you? If you don't change unhealthy lifestyle practices, your health will not improve. To paraphrase one of our greatest thinkers, Einstein, it is insanity to continue with the same actions but expect different results. But if you do make healthy changes, you will certainly feel better and you may even start feeling great.

I believe that an overburdened elimination system is the most common cause of ill health today, and the most dangerous. Fortunately, it is also treatable. In the words of one patient who once relied on laxatives (which treat only symptoms), "I have a chronic colon condition that causes a 'lazy colon.' I've spent fortunes on laxatives that really didn't work. With my doctor's permission, I started a colon cleansing program. I've been on it for seven weeks and I feel great." This patient benefited from a genuine cleansing program that addressed the causes of her ill health.

Looking at the big picture, I believe we are being cheated out of good health by ignorance. We live in a polluted environment, and our diet and lifestyle make us prone to chronic illness. Understanding that our quality of life is determined by our daily choices, we have the power to improve our health and well-being step by step. With the proper use of cleansing, we can keep our bodies healthy and vital, even as we age. Chronic ailments that are believed to be a natural part of aging can be halted in their tracks and often reversed by using health practices that take only a few moments each day. In this book, you will find simple, practical, and effective methods to help your body function as it was designed to.

Do You Need Internal Cleansing?

Our bodies perform internal cleansing on a daily, moment-by-moment basis. But our normal channels of detoxification can be overwhelmed by the polluted environment in which we live, a food supply laden with pesticides and preservatives and deficient in nutrients due to mineral-depleted soil, and an internal milieu of toxic residue caused by drugs and the by-products of a stressful life. Our natural cleansing processes need our help.

You can assist the normal cleansing process most effectively by decreasing your stress load and engaging in periodic cleansing programs (I will use the words "detoxification" and "cleansing" interchangeably in this book). Chapters 1, 4, and 5 will help you identify the keys areas of stress that contribute to failing health. Chapter 2 identifies how food and toxins are processed by your body, and chapter 3 describes the five minimum necessities for healthy bowel action. Chapter 6 discusses environmental toxins and how they affect you. Chapters 8, 9, and 10 introduce you to three cleansing programs: the first one involves food only; the second employs herbal and fiber products that can be purchased in your health food store; and the third involves a shift in what you eat, moving away from the most common food allergens while introducing scientifically formulated and proven therapeutic food powders. This third program must be carried out with the support of a licensed health care practitioner. The time it takes to complete the various recommended programs is from 2 to 8 weeks, depending on which you choose.

For those of you who want to support cleansing without engaging in a specific program, you will find recommendations throughout *Internal Cleansing*, and specifically in chapters 7, 11, 12, 13, 14, and 15. Don't feel like you have to make the time to read this book from cover to cover, though most of my patients do just that. For a quick study, read just those sections that interest you the most and come back later for the rest.

Before I explain the details of cleansing programs that I recommend, you should look over the following checklist to determine whether you would benefit from internal cleansing. Then complete the Metabolic Screening Questionnaire and the Dysbiosis Questionnaire in chapter 8 to assess your health status. These tools will give you an idea of whether you have toxic buildup in your body.

Autointoxication Checklist

If you experience any of the following symptoms, you may be experiencing autointoxication (a process whereby you are poisoned by substances produced by your own body as a result of inadequate digestion and elimination), and therefore you might want to consider some type of internal cleansing program:

- allergy or intolerance to certain foods
- bad breath and foul-smelling gas and stools
- constipation, diarrhea, sluggish elimination, irregular bowel movements
- frequent congestion, colds, viruses
- flatulence or gas and frequent intestinal disorders
- frequent headaches for no apparent reason

- general aches and pains that migrate from one place to another
- intolerance to fatty foods
- low energy, loss of vitality for no apparent reason
- lower back pain
- lowered resistance to infections
- needing to sleep a long time
- pain in your liver or gall bladder
- premenstrual syndrome (PMS), breast soreness, vaginal infections
- skin problems, rashes, boils, pimples, acne

If you have severe symptoms or any serious disorders, seek the attention of a competent health care provider. The above list is only meant to indicate some of the symptoms of autointoxication. Anyone who has been on a Standard American Diet (SAD) for more than two years would benefit from periodic cleansing, especially if you live in industrial, urban, or agricultural areas.

Please note that pregnant or lactating women should postpone their cleansing program, as toxic substances can be released to the fetus during cleansing through the shared circulation of the mother's blood or through the mother's milk. If you are pregnant or lactating, you can still help yourself and your little one by eating high-quality foods and supplementing your diet with fiber and other health promoting nutrients as described in chapter 13. Following the general rule of five servings of fruits and vegetables, one whole grain, and three high quality proteins of your choice every day will support your special needs, if combined with essential fatty acids, rest, prenatal vitamins, and an increased consumption of water (see Appendix 2).

WHERE TO START

Any cleansing program should begin by "pulling the plug" that blocks the passage of waste. The "plug" is in your colon, the last portion of your food-processing chain. If you try to clean your blood, lymph, or liver without first addressing a stopped-up large intestine, the excreted toxins will get right back into your body and make you sicker than you were before you started.

A carefully planned and monitored cleansing program will not make you sick. It has the potential to make you feel gloriously better. Sometimes just by freeing up your intestines, you can reduce the need for cleansing other circulatory or organ systems. Removing the reservoir of poisons downstream prevents them from accumulating upstream.

If you took your heart or lung cells and put them in a laboratory dish, giving the cells the food they need to live and washing away their waste products, your cells would outlive you because they would be provided with an optimum environment. When you have finished reading this book, you will have the information you need to nourish and cleanse all of your cells, thus creating a more optimal environment in order to begin a more healthful, positive way of living.

WHAT IS HEALTH COACH?

Some would have us believe that health is the mere absence of disease. The World Health Organization (WHO) defines health as the presence of complete social, mental, and physical well-being, not merely the absence of disease. Health Coach Systems International takes that definition a step farther: "Health is that state of mind, body, and spirit that allows for proper function, joy, and peace of mind." Health Coach, founded in 1991 by Mark Percival, D.C., N.D., is a group of over 200 licensed heath care practitioners in North America from various fields, who use education, inspiration, and natural therapies to help their clients and patients overcome pain, fatigue, and illness to achieve radiant health. According to Health Coach, there are four fundamental aspects of health:

1. Rest/movement/exercise
2. Eating appropriately
3. Self-reflection
4. Fun/community or loving relationships

Creating these essentials in your life is what Health Coach calls "no alternative" or self-reliant health care. No alternative simply means that there is no alternative to drinking good water, thinking good thoughts, getting rest, moving your body, eating good food, and having fun. By taking care of these fundamentals you will enjoy vibrant good health. It is interesting to note that two people with identical genetic backgrounds will enjoy different levels of health depending on how they live their lives, in other words, the lifestyle choices that they make. It's really common sense. If twins had a tendency to develop arthritis, heart disease, and senile dementia, who do you think would succumb to those diseases—the one who drinks excessive amounts of alcohol, never exercises, eats fatty red meat at practically every meal, and has a bad attitude or the one who tries to help others while making enough time to take care of him or herself, eats lots of fruits and vegetables, chooses a variety of healthy

What Determines Your Health

As you can see, your lifestyle choices are the greatest influence on your health. Education is the foundation of your health care, and with better education you make better choices.

(Reprinted by permission of Health Coach Systems International, Inc., and New Health Perspectives.)

protein sources including fish and soy products along with high quality red meat if they like, and drinks plenty of pure water? That's an easy question to answer, isn't it?

Take a moment to reflect on these four fundamentals and notice that they are influenced by your daily choices and actions. The quality of your life is determined by the quality of your choices. Of course, genetics plays a role in your health. Take a look at the chart on the previous page to see "What Determines Your Health." At the present time, it is not possible to alter your genetic makeup, but you can improve the way your genetic code expresses itself by modifying your daily lifestyle choices.

AWARENESS + ACTION = HEALTH

Health is your birthright. You can educate yourself about how your body works, and/or seek the help of a trained health professional, and begin to make wiser, health-promoting choices in the realms of eating, exercise, relaxation, and relationships, thereby leading to a happier, healthier you. But until you take action, education is worthless. To know and yet not to do is not to know. Start with some baby steps until you can take the pursuit of your health into a full-blown, joyous gallop. As British statesman and orator Edmund Burke said, "No one would make a greater mistake than he who did nothing because he could do only a little."

One of my patients remarked to me after treatment, "I have just completed six weeks of the internal cleansing program and feel better than I have in years—maybe ever! This is something I feel everyone can benefit by."

It is my hope that you, too, will feel the same way soon.

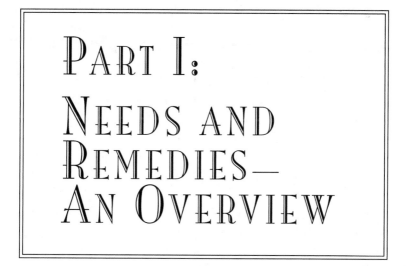

PART I:
NEEDS AND
REMEDIES—
AN OVERVIEW

CHAPTER 1

FOUR KINDS OF STRESS

Faced with adversity, human beings show an amazing ability to adapt. So why do we break down with symptoms of ill health and disease? The answer is that we encounter or endure stress greater than our bodies and minds can handle.

Four major kinds of stress lead to dysfunction, disease, and death: structural stress, biochemical stress, mental and emotional stress, and electromagnetic stress. Stress causes an accumulation of toxic substances and waste products in your system. Each thought, emotion, or physical action you take evokes a physiologic and biochemical state in your body. Toxic thoughts and emotions such as guilt, hatred, impatience, or fear create toxic chemicals with harmful effects in your body. The physical trauma of accidents or repetitive stress may result in an overproduction of internally produced chemicals that prove harmful to your system. A key Health Coach principle to keep in mind is: "The single greatest challenge your body faces is the effective management of toxins."

3

How can this be done? The main focus of this book is to offer a variety of ways to clean up the toxic waste dump that is almost certainly building up in your body with the stressors of each passing day. *Internal Cleansing* will guide you to proven and effective therapies to remove obstacles that are interfering with your effective detoxification and elimination pathways. Here you'll find simple, inexpensive, and effective procedures to decrease your toxic stress load.

To handle short-term stress situations, your body moves into an alarm state. Your adrenal glands secrete hormones that shut down the supply of blood to your gastrointestinal system and increase the supply to areas designed to get you out of danger (such as your muscles). These powerful hormones make you breathe faster and more shallowly, make your heart pump stronger and faster, and increase your sensory awareness. The long-term stress of a fast-paced life, filled with problems that nag you daily without resolution, also creates this alarm state on a chronic low-level basis. This depletes your energy and your adrenal glands, ruins your digestion, and takes a toll on your health and peace of mind. Because your body does not have the opportunity to recover between stressful moments with rest, relaxation, or exercise, you have little chance to replenish your energy reserves.

Dr. Kenneth Pelletier, a psychologist from the University of California School of Medicine in San Francisco, has found that the body cannot tell the difference between a "real" threat and an imagined one. So the potentially stressful situations that you worry about every day are as harmful to your physiology as the actual stress you face. All of these underlying worries translate into damage to your body. Japanese researchers found that mental stress changed the environment in the intestinal tract to favor the growth of pathogenic microbes at the expense of health-promoting bacteria. Why not replace worry with positive action?

More than 25 years ago, public health officials noticed an epidemic increase in the number of heart and blood-vessel diseases, which prompted an intensive search for the cause. Their discoveries placed the responsibility on dietary issues: increased intake of fat and sugar, and decreased intake of fiber. Several characteristics of the Western lifestyle were also significant factors, including a reduced level of physical exertion at work and at home, reliance on legal drugs such as alcohol and nicotine for relaxation and caffeine for a pick-me-up, and most important, the increased stresses linked to a fast-paced, ever-changing pattern of life. All of these stressors have been medically documented as contributing to a widespread increase in chronic degenerative illness and reduced overall health.

STRUCTURAL STRESS

Structural stress begins with birth. Newborns are often pulled forcibly out of the mother's womb. Some are grabbed with metal forceps or sucked out of the birth canal with a metal cap attached to the head. A cesarean delivery does not ensure a gentle birth either: The doctor pulls on the head, the shoulder—whatever can be grabbed as the baby emerges. A medical technician whom I know saw doctors in the emergency room brace their feet against the delivery table as they yanked a baby out. This is not a good beginning for your musculoskeletal and nervous systems.

Structural stress continues as you grow up and through adulthood. How many times have you fallen, been

hit with a ball, or gotten knocked down in a game of bas-
ketball, baseball, football, or volleyball? How many times
have you strained your back or the joints in your arms and
legs while playing tennis or golf, or fallen off your bicycle,
or hit the ground while rollerblading? Sports are fun, but
they can cause physical blows that lead to physical damage.
Not to mention any automobile accidents you may have
been involved in, or the injuries sustained while being a
home fix-it person. Even going to the dentist causes structural stress because of the head and mouth positions you
must maintain while having work done on your teeth and
gums. Many of my patients are coming in these days with
repetitive stress injuries from their desk jobs. Sitting and
working in a limited space and performing a limited number of motions are very confining for the body and contribute to muscular stress. Desk work may put significant
harmful strain on your lower back, wrists, hands, forearms,
shoulders, and neck.

Commonly, people are structurally stressed by the
quality of the food that they eat. A male patient in his thir-
ties came in one day complaining of pain in his back in the
area just below his shoulder blades. He had a subluxation
(misalignment) of one of the vertebra in that area, and after
a chiropractic adjustment and rubbing reflexes associated
with the small intestines that run along the bottom edge of
the ribcage, he was pain-free. I found out that he had just
returned from a trip, and the airplane food he had eaten
had not sat well in his system. As a result, the nerves in his
small intestines became irritated, which then "short-cir-
cuited" his spine and caused the misalignment. The small
intestine reflex was probably activated by congestion in his

gastrointestinal (GI) system from the less-than-optimal food he had eaten.

BIOCHEMICAL STRESS

Biochemical stress is becoming an increasingly common cause of ill health, leading to chronic ill health and death. Our government has known for a long time that we are exposed to many dangerous compounds. The U.S. government's Special Commission of 1977:369 stated, "What cannot be overlooked are the unknown consequences— among them the teratogenic and conceivably mutagenic effects—of the unremitting barrage of chemicals to which the populations of the industrialized world are subjected." (Teratogenic means "causing developmental malformations," and mutagenic means "inducing genetic mutation.") There are now over 60,000 synthetic chemicals being produced commercially, and about 1,000 newly synthesized compounds are introduced each year—that's nearly three new chemicals per day. These chemicals come in the form of drugs (over-the-counter, recreational, and prescription), food additives, pesticides, fuels, chemical fertilizers, household cleaners, glues, solvents, and by-products of industry that are released into the environment. As early as 1977, our government has been concerned about the harmful effects of man-made chemicals, but not enough has been done to protect the public.

The outside world is not the only source of toxins that disturb your health. Toxins are also produced inside your body by improper digestion of food. Before you say, "That's not me; I digest my food just fine," pause for a moment to recall if you have ever experienced gas in your intestines. Many people deal with gas on a regular basis. These gurgling and sometimes embarrassing vapors are the work of bacteria or yeasts gobbling up undigested food particles in your small and large intestines. These particles result from improper food combinations, from eating foods that your body does not agree with, and/or from eating in a rushed or agitated emotional state. (Chapter 2 examines what happens in a healthy gut and how the gut malfunctions.)

Chronically fatigued and immune-compromised people from my practice found that avoiding substances toxic to them was the most significant step they had taken to reclaim their health. (Chapters 4, 5, and 6 will help you to more clearly recognize what may be toxic to your health.) Although you cannot totally avoid environmental pollutants, you can improve your ability to transform toxins into harmless materials. These converted poisons can then be safely eliminated through your normal excretory channels of sweat, urine, feces, and breath. (Chapter 3 describes ways to enhance your ability to eliminate toxins.)

If your body cannot remove toxins through normal excretion (its first line of defense), it will step-up measures to protect itself. This is when you begin to get the "itises": colitis, sinusitis, gastritis, bronchitis, and appendicitis, to name just a few. Terms like "bronchitis," "gastritis," and others generally denote an inflammation of the part to which the ending -itis is attached. Inflammation is your body's second line of healing defense—a way of healing itself by killing off foreign invaders such as germs and allergens, diluting injurious substances such as toxins, walling off a problem area to prevent it from spreading, or simply stabilizing a weakened or injured area. When your second line of defense is ineffective at expelling waste, toxins begin to accumulate in your body in polyps, cysts, and tumors, which can progress to cancer.

ELECTROMAGNETIC STRESS

Electromagnetic stress is everywhere, from radios, televisions, cellular phones, radar, and microwaves. Young children and electrical workers are especially vulnerable to these energy frequencies. Although this is a controversial topic, research from the late 1970s through the 1990s supports a closer look at exposure to electromagnetic fields (EMFs). Metanalysis of studies reported in the medical literature from 1995 to 1999 in the United States, Germany, New Zealand, and Italy all found a risk associated with EMFs and high power lines and cancers of all types, including childhood leukemia. The metanalysis included not only exposure to high power lines but also to household EMFs.[1-4] Exposure can come from electrical appliances, including televisions (sitting too close to televisions increases your exposure to electrical radiation; protect children by making a minimum distance rule while they watch television—at least three feet from the screen), electric blankets, cooking appliances, and from electrically conductive plumbing (*Bioelectromagnetics*, 1995). Electrically conductive plumbing is found in homes whose electricity is grounded to their water pipes in an uninterrupted metallic path to the water main, which is also connected to neighboring houses. To find out if your home's electricity is grounded in this manner, you can call your local building inspector. Alternative grounding options exist. The grounding wire for your house can be connected to a nine to ten foot copper rod buried in the ground anywhere outside your home.

We are on electromagnetic overload. Mark Percival, D.C., N.D., tells about one of his patients who suffered from nightly seizures that were not relieved by medication. After carefully reviewing his case, Dr. Percival offered a number of options to decrease the stressors to this man's health and to increase his internal resilience. The patient's first steps were to increase his exposure to natural light by going outside on breaks, setting up a filter screen which reduces radiation exposure for his computer monitor, and moving his LED (light emitting diode) clock from his bedside across the room to his dresser. After only one day, this man's nighttime seizures went away. It pays to take a serious look at reducing your exposure to potentially harmful electromagnetic frequencies.

MENTAL/EMOTIONAL STRESS

At my office, we have learned to appreciate the effects of state of mind on health. Often we see patients with a pain between their shoulder blades or in the area between their neck and shoulder who have a deep anger or hurt they have been holding inside. Their pain subsides when they work through this emotion and transform it or find constructive ways to dissipate the tension they created from their repressed feelings. Anger may also cause pain and/or weakness in different parts of your body. In the Applied Kinesiology (AK) system of diagnosis and treatment (borrowing from the Chinese Five Element healing system), the pectoral muscle in your chest relates to the liver. Liver function is disturbed by anger. When people get angry they sometimes experience chest pain, which may be mistaken for a heart problem.

Knee pain may also relate to gall bladder dysfunction (the gall bladder is a small sac underneath your liver that concentrates liver secretions and releases them when the fatty foods you have eaten are in your small intestines); the popliteus muscle, which nestles into the back of your knee, is another muscle that relates to the gall bladder in the AK system. Several years ago, a woman came to my office with pain in her knees. Her mother had just died, and she was afraid that she, too, was falling apart. Upon examination, I found that the popliteus muscle behind her knee and the reflexes associated with her liver were involved. Problems in these areas can be associated with anger. I asked if she had been angry recently, and she said she had. Her mother was an alcoholic who upon her death, had left a mess of her home and her affairs, which my patient had to straighten out. She was angry at her mother for being an alcoholic, for dying from complications of alcoholism, and for leaving such a mess for her to take care of. Just knowing that her emotions were involved in her knee pain gave this patient a sense of relief. We worked on the involved areas, and she left feeling much better and had no more trouble with her knees.

Lower back pain frequently results from a disturbance of bowel function precipitated by an emotional upset or trauma. Handle the emotional upset, and the irritation carried by the nerves to the digestive organs is eliminated or decreased.

Sharon Wegscheider-Cruse, a psychologist who has been writing about dysfunctional family relationships since 1987, estimates that 96 percent of us are raised in dysfunctional families. Most of us were not raised in homes that nourished growth or supported confidence and self-esteem. Linda G. Russek and Gary E. Schwartz, in "Narrative Descriptions of Parental Love and Caring Predict Health Status in Midlife: A 35-Year Follow-Up of the Harvard Mastery of Stress Study" from the Harvard publication *Alternative Therapies* (November 1996), state: "The perception of social support is reportedly a significant predictor of future health." Students from the 1950s were asked at that time to write narrative descriptions of their parents. They found that subjects who had illnesses in mid-life such as coronary artery disease, hypertension, duodenal ulcer, and alcoholism had used significantly fewer positive words such as loving, friendly, warm, open, understanding, sympathetic, and just to describe their parents. Furthermore, 95 percent of subjects who used few positive words and who also rated their parents low in parental caring had diseases diagnosed in mid-life, whereas only 29 percent of subjects who used many positive words and also rated their parents high in parental caring had these problems. The effect was independent of the subject's age, family history of illness, smoking behavior, marital history, or the death or divorce of the subject's parents.

Emotional traumas accumulate early and may persist, leaving a person with emotional scars that get carried into adult life and relationships. To add further insult to injury, much inner dialogue is negative. In *Over the Top*, Zig Ziglar says, "The most important opinion you have is the one you have of yourself, and the most significant things you say are those things you say to yourself." One of my mentors, Charles Ward, D.C., founder of Legends in Leadership, a practice management organization, likes to remind his audience that if anyone talked to us the way we talk to ourselves we would want to get away from that person as fast as possible. Self-destructive inner dialogue may be limiting your ability to take positive steps to heal your life and your health. (For action steps you can take to resolve such internal conflicts see appendix 1.)

Stress of all kinds wears your body down and leads to an increased toxic burden in one of two ways:

1. By depleting your energy reserves and nutrients necessary for normal elimination
2. By causing an increase in toxic metabolites as a result of negative thoughts, moods and emotions, physical trauma, and impaired digestive capacity

Keep reading. You will find solutions to the problem of toxic buildup in the following pages.

CHAPTER 2

How the Body Processes Food and Toxins

The Digestion Process

In order to survive and thrive, your body must change the products you eat into microparticles, which, when absorbed, move into place to nourish your cells and become the components of your body. This process is called digestion and assimilation, or absorption. You may have heard the expression "You are what you eat." Actually, you are what you absorb. The intricate workings of your digestive system are dependent on mechanical actions such as chewing and peristalsis, and on *physiological* responses such as the secretion of enzymes. (Peristalsis is the automatic sequential contraction of the smooth muscle in your digestive tract that moves the food through the various phases of digestion from your esophagus to your rectum.) If one facet of digestion is malfunctioning, or if nutritional mediators are absent, the end products of eating become hazardous to your health, as you will learn in this chapter.

15

How Digestion Works

The chemical process of digestion begins when the thought or smell of food causes secretion of a starch-metabolizing enzyme in your saliva. Perhaps you have noticed how the simple act of talking about food can make you feel hungry.

IN THE MOUTH   Mechanical action, or chewing, is the next step. Chewing is also known as *mastication*. At the turn of the century, an American food scientist named Horace Fletcher went public with the importance of chewing. He encouraged folks to "Fletcherize" their food. The process was simple: Chew each bite about fifty times, and ingest liquids by sips.

The biochemical phase of digestion begins in earnest after mouthfuls of food have been broken down by chewing. If you gulp food down in big bites without much chewing, you put the brakes on your ability to digest food and be well-nourished because digestive juices will not come in contact with all parts of the food you have swallowed.

In the mouth, the chemical process is initiated with the release of *ptyalin,* an enzyme that begins carbohydrate (starch) digestion. You can taste the results of this enzyme's activity if you take a bite of cracker, plain bread, or plain pasta and chew it until you get a sweet taste in your mouth. A carbohydrate is made up of individual glucose (sugar) molecules. The sweet taste comes from the conversion of the starch in the cracker, bread, or pasta into simple sugars. This may be a good way for you to judge whether you are chewing your food enough: Wait until the carbohydrates in your mouth become sweet from adequate chewing before swallowing.

IN THE STOMACH   In the stomach, hydrochloric acid acts as a bulldozer and further breaks up large food particles into a semiliquid called *chyme*. Peristalsis aids the mixing of the chyme with digestive secretions to enhance the complete breakdown of food. Finally, the real digestive finesse begins: Enzymes released from the pancreas and gallbladder called amylase, lipase, and protease divide carbohydrates, fats, and proteins into simple sugars, fatty acids, and amino acids, respectively. The last phase of enzyme production is completed in the middle portion of the small intestine, called the jejunum.

IN THE SMALL INTESTINE   Absorption occurs primarily in the upper portion of the small intestine. There is, however, significant absorption of key nutrients in the colon, specifically the B-vitamins and water. When you were growing in your mother's womb, your body formed special surfaces in your intestinal tract for nutrient absorption. These surfaces are called *villi*. In the small intestine, you have even smaller finger-like projections called *microvilli* that extend into your gut lumen (the enclosed space within your intestinal tract). The microvilli are hair-like projections that carry lymphatic and blood vessels to your gut wall to interface with the partially digested food you have recently eaten (see "How Poor Digestion Affects the Lymphatic System," page 32). It takes approximately 20 minutes for food to clear your stomach and reach this digestive station. Peristaltic movement makes it possible for the chyme to wash against the absorptive surfaces of the microvilli. The two areas of your internal organs in greatest contact with the outside world are the gut lumen and the lung tissue (through the nose). They also have the highest concentration of protective immune cells in the body because both areas come in contact with potentially contaminating substances such as those found in food and in the air.

What is finally absorbed from the intricate processes of your digestive system are simple sugars from carbohydrates, amino acids from proteins, and fatty acids from fats. All of these macronutrients (proteins, carbohydrates, fats) that appear in food are essential for life. Macronutrients must be broken down into microparticles, then individual molecules, before they can be absorbed.

IN THE COLON   The colon, the last portion of your digestive system, is the final treatment area for whatever enters the digestive tract. Its job is to compact the chyme, absorb water, and receive B-vitamins that are produced by healthy intestinal bacteria. The bacteria in your intestines are tiny particles much smaller than your body's cells, and they are packed in tightly. In fact, there are more individual cells in your intestinal tract than there are known stars in the universe.

The hundred or more strains of bacteria that coexist in your intestines can be thought of as a neighborhood. There are "good guys" ready to work for your health and "bad guys" out to eat up your good nutrients, poke holes in your intestines in search of more goodies, and scavenge food that has overstayed its welcome, forming dangerous chemical by-products. These bad-guy bacteria create toxic substances that injure your intestinal wall and eventually injure your joints, skin, organs, and endocrine glands. Such everyday problems as intestinal gas and bad breath are caused by these pathogenic microorganisms, but they can also contribute to creating life-threatening diseases such as cancer.

Digestive System Breakdown

If you are under stress or in a negative state of mind when you eat, your digestive system gets a message from your nervous system to shut down and take a break because the blood and energy used for digestion are needed elsewhere. If this happens, the fat that you eat becomes rancid, the carbohydrates ferment, and the proteins putrefy. This process leads to bad breath, possibly indigestion, and altered bowel activity — either too much, causing loose stool, or too little, causing constipation. Instead of getting nutrients to feed your cells and create new ones, your cells get a serving of more waste to deal with. After a while, your cells can't handle any more waste, and they begin to break down or malfunction.

Autointoxication is the process of the body poisoning itself with toxins from internal sources that cannot be processed by the body's elimination systems because they are overloaded, undernourished, genetically compromised, or diseased. If the organs of elimination are not functioning properly, the waste matter will not be eliminated and the toxic residue will be reabsorbed into the bloodstream, causing chronic unwellness and possibly disease.

A poorly functioning digestive tract can turn even the best of foods into metabolic poisons in the form of acids, gases, alcohols, and carcinogens. This kind of digestive trouble is becoming a major source of internal toxicity in many North Americans. The fastest and surest way to detoxify your system is through improving the quality of your digestion.

HEALTH CONSEQUENCES OF INTESTINAL IRRITANTS   The presence of pathogenic organisms in the gut has been linked to arthritic disorders. As reported in the *Archives of Surgery* (December 1988), trauma, burns, chemotherapy, and inflammatory bowel disease can be related to an increase in the permeability of your bowel to microorganisms or to their endotoxins (toxic by-products). This is a condition called "leaky gut." (See appendix 4 for a test to identify this syndrome.) In the *Journal of Rheumatology* (April 1985), Smith, Gibson, and Brooks reported finding "significant alterations in bowel permeability in patients with ankylosing spondylitis (AS) and rheumatoid arthritis (RA). An association between bacterial flora in the bowel, diet, and intestinal mucosal permeability and joint disease in patients with RA and AS has been suggested by several authors, and our study further links the GI tract and inflammatory joint disease."[1]

Myasthenia gravis, a disease of the nerve/muscle junction, has been described as an *autoimmune disease,* which means that the body attacks its own cells. How does the body turn against itself? Some propose a model of infestation by pathogenic bacteria in the gut.[2] The immune system reacts to the bacterial infestation. Unfortunately, in myasthenia gravis the nerve/muscle junction looks like pathogenic bacteria to the circulating immune system cells, so they attack the vital communication link between the nervous system and muscle function.

Marjatta Leirisal-Repo, M.D., and Heikki Repo, M.D., at the Second Department of Medicine at the University of Helsinki, Finland, reported that infections of the mucosa—the lining of the inner ear and the digestive and elimination systems—can trigger the development of reactive arthritis.[3] The infection can be in the urogenital tract (the tube going from your bladder to the outside of your body) or in the gastrointestinal (GI) tract. The microbes that most frequently triggered the arthritic response were *Chlamydia, Shigella, Salmonella, Yersinia,* and *Campylobacter.* You may have heard from your doctor that the problems you were having in your elimination channels were caused by one or more of these microbes.

In an editorial by Inman in the *Journal of Rheumatology* (1987), it is learned that many gastrointestinal problems are related to arthritis.[4] People who have had intestinal bypass surgery, dysentery (Montezuma's Revenge), inflammatory bowel disease, parasites, colitis, milk allergies, and other bowel disorders have a higher incidence of arthritis than people with normal GI tracts.

What these researchers are saying is that the pain you may be experiencing in your joints could be due to a toxic bowel, to allergies, or to an autoimmune response caused by a similarity between your cells and harmful microorganisms. Internal cleansing is a possible solution to these problems (for more information, see chapters 7 and 8).

The standard medical solution for arthritis and joint pain is non-steroidal anti-inflammatory drugs (NSAIDs), such as Tylenol (acetaminophen), Advil or Motrin IB (ibuprofen), and aspirin, which are available over the counter. If NSAIDs don't relieve the pain, sometimes a medical doctor will prescribe steroids. While NSAIDs and steroids usually provide temporary relief from aches and pains, most NSAIDs inhibit the liver's ability to neutralize toxic substances, thus causing an overload of toxins in the bloodstream. Formerly injured or painful areas then become further irritated by the toxins in the blood, which in turn renews the pain cycle.

Many people notice irritation to their digestive tract when using NSAIDs. These substances can actually cause the lining of the stomach and intestines to bleed. And like antibiotics that kill off both the good and the bad bacteria, NSAIDs kill off the natural pain-relieving substances that the body produces from the good fats and oils one eats. (As a chiropractic student, I was amazed to study the effects of steroid hormones on rat joints. I can still clearly see in my mind's eye a series of photomicrographs of a normal rat joint and its appearance after only two cortisone injections. After one injection, the distinct surfaces of the joint began to break down and bleed into each other. After the second injection, the joint was completely obliterated. All of the cells had become non-distinct scar tissue instead of bone, cartilage, and synovial cells. Seeing those photos made up my mind about ever getting a steroid injection.)

If you must use NSAIDs or steroids, it is wise to use them minimally and to seek effective treatment for the cause of your pain with a respected chiropractor. Also, follow the cleansing recommendations throughout this book to minimize or eliminate the inflammatory agents that trigger joint destruction.

Food and Health

Five major or *macronutrient* categories are required for life: water, proteins, carbohydrates, fats, and fiber. The current craze for a high protein, low carbohydrate, low-fat diet is not compatible with human physiology. We need approximately 20 to 30 percent good fats, 20 to 30 percent protein, and 40 to 60 percent carbohydrates.

Because we are all biochemically unique, we each need different proportions of fats, protein, and carbohydrates. Depending on what is happening in your life, your individual needs also change. If your diet consists mostly of refined carbohydrates such as pasta, crackers, and bread, you are creating an imbalance in your body that promotes fat storage, increases pain, suppresses your immune system, depletes your hormones, destabilizes your cell membranes, and places strain on your heart and blood vessels. Likely outcomes of this kind of diet include obesity; muscle and joint pain; increased susceptibility to infection, common colds, and flu; infertility, impotency, and menstrual difficulties; wrinkles, dry skin, and acne; and heart attacks and blood vessel disease.

The Vicious Cycle of Food Hypersensitivity

Many people were fed food other than mother's milk as an infant, before their digestive tract had completely formed. In such people there is a high probability of food hypersensitivities. Think about the foods that babies are typically fed: cow's milk and related dairy products, cereal grains (especially wheat), eggs, citrus, and soy-based products. These are the most common food *allergens* (substances that cause a hypersensitive or allergic reaction). The high incidence of childhood ear infections (treated by one antibiotic after another and too often culminating in surgery to insert plastic tubes into the ears of preschool-age children) is probably the result of food hypersensitivities (see appendix 1).

To add to your digestive confusion, grains have only been a part of the human diet for the past ten thousand years. That is a long time compared with the human life span, but a very short time compared with the length of time that humans have inhabited the Earth. In most native cultures people who eat grains sprout them before eating to make them more digestible and culture milk products before use for the same reason. Other causes of food allergies include weakened adrenal glands from too much stress and inadequate time spent resting, relaxing, and exercising; a weak or impaired digestive system from drugs including over-the-counter NSAIDs, alcohol, antibiotics, excess sugar, preservatives, pesticides, and food additives; lack of variety in the diet, or eating the same foods over and over; and a deficiency of digestive enzyme secretion by your body, perhaps from unrelenting stress.

If you are eating foods to which you are hypersensitive, you may suffer from fatigue, heart palpitations, insomnia, indigestion, the full component of digestive disturbances, frequent illnesses, confusion, mental disorders, body aches, and pains; anything can go wrong. For example, people who are sensitive to gluten (found in wheat and other grains except rice) but eat gluten-containing foods anyway have a much higher incidence of dementia than people without this sensitivity. At a Health Coach Retreat called "Physician Heal Thyself," doctors and their support staffs reintroduced foods after eliminating major food allergens for a six-day period and eating a simple diet. Reactions to foods on reintroduction included anxiety from eating an egg; unrelenting diarrhea, an upper respiratory infection, and depression from eating wheat; burning pain running down the backs of both arms and legs from eating tomatoes; depression from eating brown rice; and lethargy from eating millet. If you eat a food to which you are hypersensitive every day, you won't have such a pronounced reaction. Instead of getting an acute attack of sickness, you will be chronically unwell; your body adapts to the substance.

STEROID USE AND FOOD HYPERSENSITIVITIES If you have a history of using antibiotics, steroids, synthetic hormones (such as birth control pills), or cortisone and its medical relatives—or even if you have drunk chlorinated water—the chances are good that you have an imbalance of intestinal microorganisms, with the bad guys outweighing the good guys. When this happens, the pathogenic yeasts or bacteria may invade or irritate your intestinal wall, causing damage that leads to a leaky gut (see appendix 4). The leaky gut allows big molecules of food to pass through your intestinal wall and enter your bloodstream. Your immune system is then put on alert and mobilizes lymphocytes, macrophages, and other natural killer cells to protect you against these foreign invaders to your bloodstream. An inflammatory cascade ensues, which may lead to colitis, irritable bowel syndrome, sinusitis, arthritis, or any other "-itis" you can imagine.

How do you determine which foods you are sensitive to? When you react to foods, two main types of antibodies are produced: immunoglobulins E and G (IgE and IgG, respectively). IgE antibodies are fast acting and cause an almost immediate response, which is why traditional allergists check for them. Unfortunately, most of us have delayed negative reactions to foods, which may take up to 4 days to appear. This delay makes it hard to track what caused the problem or to even determine that foods are linked to health complaints. For instance, I have a delayed sensitivity reaction to caffeine. It takes almost 2 days before I get a headache from coffee. Throughout chiropractic school, I drank coffee to help me meet the demands of my rigorous schedule, and I suffered headaches on a regular basis. When I got into practice, I wanted to be a good example to my patients, so I stopped drinking coffee except after lunch, when I attended educational seminars. That cup of coffee helped me stay awake for the afternoon sessions. I finally realized that the headaches I was getting almost 2 days later were reactions to the caffeine. IgG antibodies mediate this kind of hypersensitivity. To help their patients better, many healthcare practitioners on the vanguard of healing practices recommend that their patients be tested for both kinds of antibodies with an ELISA test (ELISA tests are blood tests that help you and your doctor identify both immediate and delayed hypersensitivity reactions).

A less expensive but more complex method of testing for allergies and hypersensitivities is elimination and provocation. In this process, you eliminate the most common allergens, including gluten-containing products (e.g., wheat in all its forms), citrus fruit, beef, peanuts, soy, and dairy products. After 2 to 3 weeks, you add these foods back to your diet one at a time and observe your physical and emotional reactions. Anything out of the ordinary or a return of a symptom that had been absent during the elimination phase is a sure sign that the recently reintroduced food is not good for you at the present time.

Dr. Peter D'Adamo, a naturopathic physician, correlates foods that are beneficial, neutral, and harmful to patients depending on their blood type. Although no one system has the answer for everyone, I find it useful for myself and my patients to avoid the foods designated as harmful. Some people may find that foods recommended as beneficial may cause problems. We are all biochemically unique. Unfortunately, there are no "one size fits all" programs. If you would like to know more about Dr. D'Adamo's program, check out his Web site www.dadamo.com.

How Food Combining Affects Digestion

Some nutrition experts emphasize combining your food properly to solve digestive upset. In brief, because of enzyme action, you digest your food more easily if you avoid eating starches and proteins in combination. (John Montague, Fourth Earl of Sandwich, started a lot of trouble with his eighteenth-century invention of putting meat between two slices of bread.) Most meals are nightmares of bad food combining; consider the Standard American Diet:

- Breakfast—Orange juice with simple sugars; toast, usually a refined carbohydrate with little fiber; eggs, a protein; and bacon, a protein fat food full of carcinogenic nitrosamines.
- Lunch—A sandwich or a burger consisting of starch and meat protein.
- Dinner—Meat with potatoes or rice, and a sugary dessert.

Eating this way causes several days' worth of meals to back up in your intestines (Figure 2.1). No wonder Americans have such upset stomachs!

If you have digestive complaints, first try eating your food in a more relaxed state of mind. Take some deep breaths and feel your belly expand before you begin eating. Put your fork down between bites, and spend more time enjoying your food. Regardless of what you eat, this simple step will improve your digestion immensely. But if it doesn't help enough, you might want to experiment with eating less food at one time or by following basic food-combining principles. When you eat high-starch vegetables, combine them only with high-water-content vegetables (see Carbohydrate

Food transit time of person on a Standard American Diet (low fiber) diet. Average transit time is 65–100 hours.

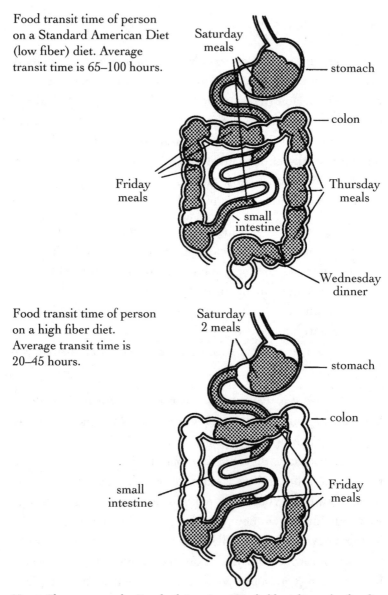

Food transit time of person on a high fiber diet. Average transit time is 20–45 hours.

NOTE: The person on the Standard American Diet holds eight meals of undigested food and waste material in the colon, while the person on the high fiber diet holds only three.

Figure 2.1   Food Transit Times

Classifications of Fruits and Vegetables charts in chapter 8). When you eat protein, combine it only with high-water-content vegetables. In practice, if you eat the bread that is served before your meal in a restaurant, you should choose a vegetable meal and eat your protein at a later time. Or avoid eating the bread and eat only the vegetables and protein on your plate, but not the rice or potatoes. I often ask for a double portion of vegetables instead of the starch on the menu when I eat a protein meal out. You may benefit from doing the same if you have digestive difficulties.

Another food combining principle is to eat melons alone, not in combination with any other food. If you love melons, you could eat more food 20 to 30 minutes later when the melon has cleared your stomach.

I find that my digestive system gets in an uproar if I eat raw fruit and raw vegetables at the same meal. Your digestive system is unique. Only by trial and error will you find the right food combinations. Remember: Awareness + Action = Health.

How Hormones Affect Digestion and Elimination

To have a healthy digestive tract, you must also have a properly functioning thyroid gland. Thyroid hormones help your intestines with peristalsis; if you have a sluggish thyroid, you will probably have a sluggish bowel, causing chronic constipation and the subsequent backup of toxins into your blood. Unfortunately, current blood tests for thyroid function tell us only the amount of thyroid hormone in your blood; they cannot tell us whether the hormone is getting into your cells and working where it's supposed to.

Thyroid blood tests are unreliable because we can't get information on the functional capacity of the thyroid from blood tests. Dr. Broda O. Barnes developed a protocol for evaluating the function of the thyroid gland by measuring underarm temperature before you get out of bed in the morning. You can now do this test with a digital thermometer. Make sure you do nothing more than reach with your arm for the thermometer before you take your temperature. If you sit up and lean on your elbow, your temperature will elevate. Record the temperature before you get out of bed. Follow this procedure for at least six mornings in a row to get the best information. If you are a menstruating woman, your temperature will rise around the time of ovulation because of a hormone surge, so it is best to avoid taking readings mid-cycle. The normal range for resting temperature is 97.8 to 98.2 degrees F. If your temperature is below 97.8 degrees F, you have a low-functioning thyroid (hypothyroid). According to the Dr. Broda O. Barnes Foundation, hypothyroid people will exhibit any one of more than 100 symptoms, and no two people will have the same symptoms. However, some overt signs of a low-functioning thyroid include fatigue, constipation, cold hands and feet, dry skin, loss of the outer third of the eyebrow, hyperlaxity of joints (being double-jointed), and backward-facing palms when standing.

Some people need prescription thyroid medication to boost their levels of thyroid hormone. Most medical doctors have been trained to prescribe Synthroid, which needs to be split by liver enzymes before it can work in the cell. Mercury and other toxins may inhibit the enzyme from being able to activate the Synthroid at the cellular level. In addition, the receptor sites for the hormones on your cells can get filled up by mercury and other toxic substances, preventing the thyroid hormone from binding to your cells and stimulating normal functions such as an increased basal metabolic rate and increased energy production. Whole-gland prescription medications such as Armour Desiccated Thyroid and Naturthroid may be helpful. The already acti-vated form of thyroid called Cytomel may also be helpful. You will need to work with a trained physician to find the right kind and dose of thyroid for you. There are now blood tests for free thyroid hormones (T3 and T4), which check for the active form of the hormones. It still can't tell us whether the cells are being activated by the free hormone but it gets us closer than before to information regarding thyroid function. (See appendix 1.)

As we have seen, toxicity is a major cause of this mal-function of thyroid stimulation in your cells. Cleansing will help every cell of your body function at a higher level of performance, making you think, feel, and look better. It makes sense to start a quality detoxification program before taking prescription medication. It may be all that your body needs to get you back on track to good health.

Dr. Joseph and Mary Ann Mayo, who are authors of the helpful book *The Menopause Manager,* find that gut func-tion is powerfully affected by a woman's sex hormones and sex hormones are powerfully affected by gut toxicity. Mary Ann, a psychotherapist who works closely with her hus-band, stated, "In our clinical experience at our former clinic A Woman's Place Medical Center, it was clear that the ma-jority of our patients could benefit by some form of improve-ment to gut function. Specifically, we found that patients who underwent a gut detoxification program found that their need for menopausal intervention (including drug ther-apy) was reduced and/or that the interventions they used worked more effectively. It is important that menopausal symptoms due to hormone readjustment be distinguished from symptoms due to poor gut health. Too often mid-life women assume everything they are experiencing is due to menopause."

How Poor Digestion Affects the Lymphatic System

Let's now consider the job of the lymphatic vessels teamed up with the blood vessels in your villi, which are designed to protect your body from harmful microbes. In response to a pathogen, your lymph vessels release fighter lymphocytes to protect your body from being invaded. If you have a well-balanced mind and body, the immune system releases just the right amount of protector cells and natural killer cells to do the job, but if your system is under stress and overburdened with toxins and a diet that causes hypersensitivity reactions, it will surely overreact. The degree of overreaction depends on the extent of your body's overload. The hyper-response may cause a generalized inflammatory reaction in your GI tract, disturbing your ability to absorb nutrients and initiating an inflammatory cascade that may also affect distant parts of your body. Hence, you can get musculoskeletal pain as a result of a germ. Most people can relate to this problem, having experienced soreness and achiness with a cold or flu. Chronic musculoskeletal pain may be related to a chronic imbalance of good versus bad microbes in your GI tract. Lean back in your chair and press into your abdomen from your rib cage down to your pubic bone and all the way out to the sides as well. Are there any sore spots? If so, you have inflammation in your gastrointestinal tract. Periodic cleansing programs are the perfect remedy for such ills.

When you consume more fat in a meal than your body can effectively metabolize (like most Americans do), the excess is swept into the lymph vessels and circulated until your fat digesters can handle more, or it gets stored in fat cells. The Inuit Eskimos of northern Canada eat the fat of sea mammals and fish whose fat stores toxic residues. Along with the fat, the Inuit consume the toxic products of industrial pollution. (Read more about their plight in chapter 6.) Toxins get stored in the fat of all plants and animals, so even if you aren't eating whale blubber for dinner, you are being exposed to pollution particles from what you eat. These damaging particles can wreak havoc within your immune system, causing damage to cells and a hyperimmune protective response. But while the toxins in fat may cause a hyperimmune response, the presence of excess fat suppresses the ability of your immune system to respond to germs, leaving you more susceptible to infections, colds, and flus. And even if your lymph is activated to react to the toxins in the fat, it may not have the ability to respond to harmful microorganisms.

If your lymph system is congested, you will probably feel enlarged lymph nodes or glands. A good place to check for enlarged lymph nodes and glands is under your jaw and in the area between the corners of your jaw and your ear. Press up with your fingers; if these glands are tender, you are probably dealing with an acute infection. If they are swollen but not tender, it may be chronic. Other areas to check for lymph node congestion are at the crease of your leg in the groin area, in your armpits, and along the muscles in the front of your neck and at the base of your skull. A word of caution: Sometimes lymph node enlargement is associated with diseases of the lymphatic system and should be checked by your medical doctor. If you do not have a disease, there are suggestions for clearing lymph congestion in chapter 11.

Elimination via the Skin

Your largest organ of elimination is your skin. It is designed by nature to excrete bodily wastes through your pores and sweat glands. It is essential to let your body perspire, for the sake of your skin and your whole body. In fact, some detoxification strategies are designed around sweating. Historically, people have used saunas, sweat lodges, and steam baths to purify their bodies.

Dr. William Rea of Dallas, Texas, developed a "cleansing through sweating" protocol designed around moderate exercise, nutritional supplementation—particularly niacin, one of the B-vitamins—and sweating in a low-temperature sauna. The minimum amount of time needed to initiate the cleansing process is 2 weeks, but he encourages his patients to continue with the cleansing protocols at home on a regular basis. This type of program has tremendous results, particularly in detoxifying people who have a history of anesthesia or prescribed or recreational drug use (see appendix 1 for info on how to contact Dr. Rea's clinic).

If you have an overload of toxins in your body, you may notice the result as unpleasant skin conditions. One patient had skin problems until she began internal cleansing: "A severe rash on my elbows and forearms that I had for many years is clearing up and is almost gone." The importance of the skin and cleansing protocols is discussed in more detail in chapter 15.

How the Liver and Kidneys Nourish and Detoxify

The liver and kidneys filter blood and have the challenging task of distinguishing between unwanted toxins and needed nutrients. The kidneys conserve water and balance electrolytes by reabsorbing the exact amounts required minute by minute and sending the excess out through the urinary tract. This is done via a sophisticated network of electrochemical responses, including the brain, nervous system, and endocrine (hormone-producing) glands. If you have been eating a diet high in refined carbohydrates and sugar, and low or deficient in good fats, your body simply won't have the raw material available to make the hormones it needs.

The liver is a complex organ that both stores nutrients and detoxifies the bloodstream. All blood that leaves the intestines goes through the liver first before it is sent out to the rest of your body. Your liver acts as a shield to ensure that harmful substances absorbed through your gut wall are made safe or stored in a relatively non-active fatty tissue. NSAIDs inhibit the liver's ability to detoxify; the body's safety net is breached, and the floodgates are left open for damaging substances to harm your every cell.

One of the functions of the liver is to deconjugate, or break down, hormones. If the liver is damaged by excess fat, toxins, drugs, or alcohol, you can end up with too many hormones in your bloodstream. This is a major factor in premenstrual syndrome (commonly known as PMS). The hormones involved in the menstrual cycle are hydrophilic, or water loving, and cause bloating even in the brain, which creates some of the emotional tension that women may feel before and during menstruation. An excess of hormones in the bloodstream may also contribute to the increasing incidence of cancer in both men's and women's sex glands because of overstimulation. Women who have a longer exposure to their own estrogen through more frequent menstrual periods and a higher total number of menstrual cycles have a higher incidence of breast, ovary, uterine, and neck cancers.

Look for these signs and symptoms of liver distress:

- acne and other skin disorders
- inability to digest fats, which may show up as nausea or light-colored stools
- constipation or diarrhea
- pain between your shoulder blades, especially on your right side
- pain in your muscles between the neck and shoulder
- headaches, especially ones that begin in the neck/shoulder area and travel up the side of your head, around your ear, and into your eye
- anger and irritability
- multiple allergies/sensitivities

Blood tests can reveal liver pathology, but a simple at-home test can help you determine whether you would benefit from liver cleansing: Lie on your back with your knees bent and your feet flat. Place the fingers of both hands at the edge of your rib cage on the right side on a line directly below your nipple. Inhale deeply and as you exhale press your fingers firmly up under your rib cage in the direction of your head.

If this pressure causes pain—especially if it makes you draw your breath in sharply and stop breathing—you should consult a trained health-care professional who can guide you in a liver cleansing program. If you have discomfort but not pain, you would be wise to engage in some of the cleansing suggestions recommended in the following chapters and take a look at what you can change in your lifestyle to decrease your toxic load.

CHAPTER 3

Natural Elements of a Clean Bowel

Perhaps the most frequently reported bowel problem that people experience is constipation. Constipation is commonly related to a low-fiber diet, which causes fecal matter to become condensed and compressed. Evacuation then becomes infrequent and difficult. There are five major factors to consider when you have sluggish elimination from your bowel. We will investigate each of these five areas briefly:

1. Are you getting enough fiber in your diet?
2. Are you drinking adequate amounts of pure water?
3. Does your diet include high-quality essential fatty acids?
4. Do you pay attention when nature calls?
5. Do you get enough exercise?

In the past decade, the terms "constipated" and "regularity" have been redefined by medical research. A *constipated* system is one in which the transition time of toxic waste matter is slow and the consistency of the stool causes strain. The longer the transit time, the longer the toxic waste matter sits in the bowel, allowing proteins to putrefy, fats to become rancid, and carbohydrates to ferment. The longer your body is exposed to rotting food in your intestines, the greater your risk of developing disease. Even with one bowel movement per day, you still have at least three meals' worth of waste sitting in your colon most of the time.

During evacuation, hard stools place a strain on the colonic muscles and on the lining of the lower portion of your large intestine, rectum, and anus. Straining contributes to the formation of hemorrhoids, varicose veins, hiatal hernia, and a host of other mechanically induced problems. Your system can also become polluted by poisonous gases caused by stagnation in your bowel. These gases can enter your bloodstream, irritating your organs and joints. Alternating constipation and diarrhea or diarrhea alone are also indications of foulness in your intestines. Finally, the much more serious and life-threatening problems of cancer and immune system disorders may begin inside a toxic bowel. I will recommend effective strategies for overcoming these health challenges throughout *Internal Cleansing*.

Recently, two patients came to my office suffering with serious constipation. One was having, at best, five bowel movements per week. The other said he had eliminated only once every 4 days since he was a small boy. Perhaps your intestines have a similar rhythm of malfunction, and perhaps your medical doctor—like that of the first patient—has told you that this level of excretion is okay. Her doctor's perspective was that some people just have fewer bowel movements than others. That is true, but what he neglected to tell her is that those who have fewer bowel movements are harboring a breeding ground for disease and death.

After reading this book, you will understand why infrequent bowel movements are dangerous to your health. Once you have learned, please advise others who have slow-moving bowels about the importance of effectively eliminating waste products from the intestinal tract. Dr. Anthony Bassler, a gastroenterologist, says to his colleagues, "Every physician should realize that the intestinal toxemias are the most important primary and contributing causes of many disorders and diseases of the human body."

Let's take a look at what happens to the shape of your lower intestines when toxic matter has built up on your intestinal walls for years (Figure 3.1). When the colon becomes impacted with dry putrefactive waste, its shape and function are affected in many ways. It will stretch like a balloon in certain areas, or develop diverticula (pouches on the intestinal wall), or fall upon itself (a condition called prolapsus). All of these malformations greatly impair your large intestine's ability to function, which in turn places severe strain on your digestive organs and glands.

Frequently, lower back pain, neck and shoulder pain, wrist and hand pain, skin problems, "brain fog," fatigue, sluggishness, and colds and flus are caused by a blocked or slow-moving bowel. Even the common headache can be attributed to bowel dysfunction. Neurological problems are made worse by toxicity. A male patient in his fifties who has an abnormal walk due to a disc problem in his neck found that he walked better and felt more balanced after doing an internal cleansing program designed for his particular needs.

Normal colon   Ballooned sigmoid

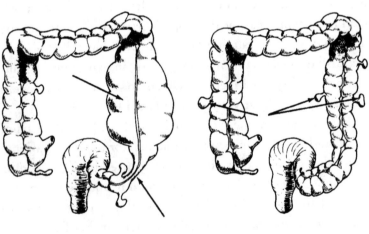

Colitis   Diverticula

Figure 3.1   Colon Dysfunctions.

Reprinted, by permission, from *Tissue Cleansing Through Bowel Management* by Dr. Bernard Jensen.

Spasm

Stricture

Prolapsus

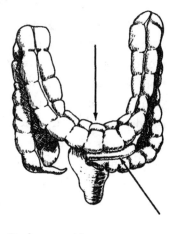

Prolapsus with pressure
on lower organs

Figure 3.1 (continued)

THE ROLE OF FIBER
IN INTESTINAL HEALTH

In August of 1984, the National Cancer Institute issued a statement called "Dietary Fiber and Lower Colon Cancer Risk," which states: "Research data suggesting that fiber-containing foods provide some protection against colon and rectal cancer have led the National Cancer Institute to make recommendations now that Americans eat a diet high in fiber from whole grain breads and cereals and fresh fruits and vegetables. If followed, these recommendations may reduce individual risk of these cancers." The statement goes on to affirm that "basic relationships between intake of fiber-containing foods and human cancer are now firmly established in the scientific literature."

On average, Americans get only about 15 grams, half the fiber necessary, every day. A shocking 25 percent of Americans get only five to seven grams per day or less. No wonder there are so many digestive problems in our population, or that $700 million worth of laxatives are sold every year. No wonder so many of us suffer with hemorrhoids, appendicitis, ulcerative colitis, diverticular disease, adenomatous polyps (considered to be early markers of colon cancer development), colon cancer, and heart disease.

Denis P. Burkitt, M.D., a physician who worked extensively with native peoples in Africa, wrote about the link between low-fiber diets and increased risk of modernization diseases in his landmark December 1969 article in *The Lancet*, a peer-reviewed medical journal. He noted that the conditions listed previously were "exceedingly rare" in rural Africa. However, as their diets became more Western (see the Standard American Diet in chapter 4) with decreased amounts of fiber, increased amounts of refined carbohydrates, in particular white flour products, and increased amounts of fat, the rural Africans experienced a rise in the incidence of these troubling conditions and life-threatening diseases.[1] In the United States, more than 19 percent of calories come from products containing bleached white flour.

Because a lack of fiber causes slower movement of feces through your bowel, it allows carcinogenic substances to be in contact with your intestinal wall longer. This could lead to possible formation of colon cancer (see Figure 3.2 for the beneficial properties of fiber).

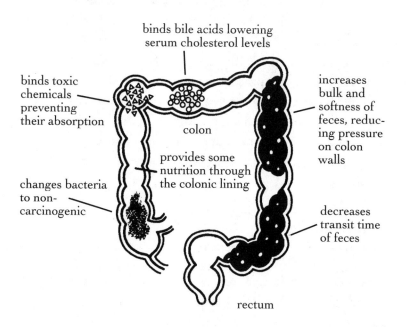

Figure 3.2   The Protective Properties of Fiber

Fiber and Lignins

Fiber also provides nutrition to your bowel flora — the friendly microorganisms in your intestines that work to promote your health. If these bacteria are fed well with certain types of plant fibers they reproduce in greater numbers and produce a substance called mammalian lignan, which increases your resistance to infectious agents and cancer. Plant fibers are the preferred source of food for your friendly bacteria. They will convert to taking in nutrients from the bowel only during times of fasting or starvation.

The fiber in flaxseed generates one hundred times more lignans than any other fiber source. (Flaxseed is one of the best sources of essential fatty acids; see "Essential Fatty Acids" later in this chapter.) Breast cancer patients, and others at high risk for colon and breast cancer, excrete far fewer lignans than healthy people. This implies that they have fewer lignans present in their bowel than do people without these types of cancers. To decrease your risk of getting breast or colon cancer, include fresh ground flaxseed — also called flax meal — in your diet on a regular basis.

For more information on dietary fiber, please see chapter 7.

THE ROLE OF WATER IN INTESTINAL HEALTH

If you do not drink enough water, your body will dry out and it will be difficult to have a bowel movement. It is impossible to overstate the importance of pure water. Your body is mostly water — 50 to 75 percent. You will absorb some water through your skin by soaking in a bathtub or by swimming, but your main source is, of course, drinking water. You need to drink water because every day you lose water through sweat, urine, and breath.

How many glasses of water do you drink each day? Many people are so out of touch with sufficient water consumption that they don't even know they are thirsty; they have suppressed their internal message to rehydrate by making the busywork of life a priority over taking care of their basic health needs. Generally, six to eight glasses (eight ounces per glass) of water per day is recommended for the average adult. However, for detoxification purposes you will need more water (see chapter 13 for specific quantities).

The quality of your health is directly related to the quality of your drinking water (see chapter 6 to learn about water quality standards). Most importantly, drink pure water on a daily basis for your best health. (For further discussions on water consumption, the environment, and filtration, see chapters 5 and 6.)

ESSENTIAL FATTY ACIDS

Essential fatty acids (EFAs) play a role in hormone and immune system function, both of which are critical to bowel health. They provide the raw materials from which your body produces hormones. EFAs also provide for the smooth functioning of your immune system for the free flow of blood through your arteries and veins, forming sheaths around your nerves to protect the integrity of information transmission along your nerves. Your hormones, immune system, vascular system (arteries and veins), and nervous system all coordinate to ensure a healthy bowel. Hormones activate movement in your intestinal muscles to aid digestion and elimination. Your immune system protects the rest of your body from invasion by toxic substances and pathogenic microorganisms that can otherwise pass from your bowel into your body. Your immune system also regulates the amount of inflammation in your intestines. Your arteries and veins supply nourishment to the cells that line your intestines and take away toxic metabolites. Your nerves command the function of every cell in your body, including your intestines, and carry information on the status of your bowel back to your brain so it knows what to do to regulate normal function. (See appendix 3 for more information on EFAs.)

As their name implies, EFAs are essential to human health. According to Edward Siguel, M.D., in his book *Essential Fatty Acids in Health and Disease,* "Without essential fats, cells do not work, organs die prematurely, brain function deteriorates."[2] In nutritional literature, nutrients are called "essential" because your body cannot make them; you must get them from your diet or from nutritional supplements.

When I review a list of all of the food, condiments, and beverages my patients have consumed for a week, I find that 100 percent of the time they are either deficient or totally lacking in EFAs. Experts agree that a diet deficient in EFAs is hazardous to your health. Your body is made up of 100 trillion cells, and every cell needs EFAs to make its cell wall and to burn for energy. The gray matter in the human brain is 50 percent EFAs. Infants and young children are especially vulnerable to EFA deficiency states because their brains and bodies are developing and adding mass. If EFAs are not available from their mothers' milk or in their diet, normal brain, nervous system, immune system, and heart development will not occur.

The recommended quantity of EFA supplementation is one teaspoon of flaxseed oil per day for each 35 pounds of body weight. As indicated by the following chart, a person weighing between 105 and 139 pounds would need to consume up to four teaspoons of flaxseed oil per day to achieve and maintain optimal health (three teaspoons equal one tablespoon).

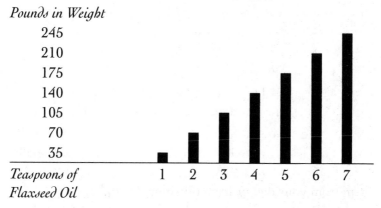

Flaxseed Oil Recommendations

Two important classes of EFAs are *omega-3* and *omega-6*. Omega-3 EFAs can be found in reliable quantities in flaxseed oil and fresh water fish. They can be found in small amounts in pumpkin seeds and walnuts. It is important to take in these nutrients in a healthy balance. Unfortunately, the type of diet we eat today supplies only one-eighth of the omega-3 content of the traditional hunter/gatherer diet, which helped us evolve into beings with a large brain-to-body ratio. To further complicate your omega-3 deficiency, modern food processing and lifestyles create *antinutrients* that call for even higher doses of omega-3 EFAs to balance their toxic effects. These antinutrients include:

- Saturated fat in the form of commercially-raised animal fats from meat, eggs, full-fat dairy products, and the skin of poultry.
- Altered fats called *trans fatty acids* in margarine and other hydrogenated, partially hydrogenated, and fractionated vegetable oils commonly found in chips, crackers, salad dressings, icings, candy bars, and baked goods (health-food-store candy is frequently made with partially fractionated palm kernel oil—an especially damaging trans fat).
- Peanut butter, peanuts, and peanut oil.
- Refined sugar and flour.
- Processed foods (Dr. Donald Rudin and Clara Felix say that, before supermarket food reaches your plate, it may have been acidified, antibiotically treated, antioxidated, artificially colored, artificially flavored, artificially supplemented, broiled/boiled, bromated, chemically enriched, chlorinated, defatted, defibered, dehydrated, emulsified, fried, hybridized, hydrogenated, marbled, nitrated, phosphated, salted, and/or sugared; see appendix 3 for information on their books).
- Caffeine, alcohol, and cigarettes.
- Recreational, prescription, and over-the-counter drugs.

For better health, minimize saturated animal fat in your diet and balance what you do eat with sources of omega-3 EFAs. If you have arthritis or other inflammatory conditions, you may see improvements if you eliminated the saturated animal fat altogether. Throw out any trans fatty acids and minimize eating out because restaurant food is loaded with trans fats. Peanut butter should not be eaten by anyone with an inflammatory condition because it promotes pain and swelling. Refined sugar and flour are not good for you, but if you do eat them, make up for it by eating more fruits and vegetables. Processed food and cigarettes only do harm. Caffeine and alcohol in small amounts are okay if you insist on using them. As for drugs of all sorts, seek alternatives first and use only as a final option.

Our ancestors got their omega-3 EFAs from fish, shellfish, and mollusks; land and water plants; nuts and seeds; and wild game. Examine your own diet to see how much high-quality food of this nature you eat on a daily basis. Today grass fed beef and lamb can substitute for wild game. Omega-6 EFAs come from warm weather oils such as safflower, canola, and soybeans and in the seeds and oils of sesame, sunflower, walnut, and pumpkin. They are essential, but more readily available in the American diet, though some may need to supplement with these oils as well. In order for the omega-3 fatty acids to perform their vital functions, other essential nutrients (proteins, vitamins, and minerals) must be present in your diet in adequate amounts. And substances antagonistic to EFAs must be eliminated or dramatically reduced. (See appendix 3 for more information.)

Americans have been concerned about reducing the quantity of fats and oils they consume. Despite their efforts, however, 30 percent more Americans are obese now than in 1970. How can that be? Many in the nutritional field attribute this trend at least partially to the reduction or elimination of EFAs from our diets. Udo Erasmus, in *Fats That Heal, Fats That Kill*, states, "[EFAs] stimulate metabolism, increase metabolic rate and oxidation, and speed up the rate at which our bodies burn fats and glucose when they get more than 12 to 15 percent of total calories as EFAs. In these quantities (upwards of three tablespoons per day), EFAs burn off excess fat and help a person to lose weight and stay slim."[3] In *The Facts About Fats*, John Finnegan describes the experience of people who added EFAs to their daily diet: "Many of my friends and clients report that, after adding in one to two tablespoons a day of flaxseed oil to their diets, they have lost their cravings for fatty foods and have experienced continued weight loss, increased energy, and a sense of dietary satisfaction."[4]

This happy occurrence is brought to us by EFAs' regulation of *brown fat*, a metabolically active form of fat that maintains body temperature by burning calories. Brown fat is concentrated around the spine and organs.

TRANS FATTY ACIDS

A discussion of trans fatty acids (TFAs) is warranted here. TFAs cause damage to your cells. They interfere with and inhibit all of the functions of omega-3 EFAs. TFAs dramatically increase the amount of toxins your body must deal with, inhibiting cleansing and destroying health (see Figure 3.3). TFAs are produced by current food processing techniques, primarily a process called hydrogenation. In order to increase shelf life and increase the marketability of oil, modern food technology experts violated the healthy chemical configuration of vegetable oils. In his book, *The Facts About Fats*, John Finnegan notes, "The effects of poorly processed oils are a major factor in heart disease, cancer and most modern diseases that have affected hundreds of millions of people all over the world."[5]

cis fatty acid
The Hs are on the same side
of the double bond, forcing
the molecule to assume
horseshoe shape.

trans fatty acid
The Hs are on opposite sides
of the double bond, forcing
the molecule into an
extended position.

Figure 3.3   Cis vs. *Trans* Fatty Acid Configuration

Nature provides us with vegetable oils in a chemical form called the *cis* configuration. The form provided to us in nature is biologically active, meaning that your body can break it down into its tiny constituents and make it into "you." The *trans* form made by man is not biologically active, meaning that you have been unknowingly cheating your body of needed nutrition when you eat a trans fat.

The most common source of these trans fats is margarine. The public has been led to believe that margarine will protect them from developing heart disease. Unfortunately, the reverse is true. Eating margarine and other forms of trans fats will increase your risk of death by heart disease. Researchers believe this happens because the altered oil damages your cells and robs them of the nutrients needed to protect you from chronic degenerative diseases. Altered oils and the deficiency of EFAs have been implicated not only in the causation of heart disease but also in such health conditions as:

- Inflammatory conditions such as colitis, diverticulitis, sinusitis, gingivitis, gastritis, and arthritis
- Immune system dysfunction
- Hormone regulation problems including PMS, menstrual cramps, infertility, impotence, vaginal dryness, and prostate enlargement
- Allergic disorders
- Crohn's Disease
- Retinal blindness
- Diabetes
- Skin disorders such as acne; eczema; psoriasis; seborrheic dermatitis; dandruff; dry, cracked and scaling skin; sun sensitivity; sudden hair loss in defined patches; and rough, prickly skin on the upper arms, elbows, thighs, and buttocks
- Childhood problems such as Sudden Infant Death Syndrome (SIDS), Attention Deficit Hyperactivity Disorder (ADHD), autism, and dental problems
- Manic depressive disorder, anxiety, schizophrenia, and agoraphobia
- Aging: wrinkles, age spots, graying hair, glaucoma

In order to get the highest quality oils, buy those that are organic and have been processed in the absence of light and air with presses of a size that you can get your arms around. Refer to the list of resources in appendix 1 for a listing of these suppliers.

To enjoy the benefits of EFAs, build your diet around plenty of omega-3 and omega-6 EFAs. Food sources of these essential healing oils are cold water fish, including salmon, mackerel, cod, and halibut; walnuts, flaxseed, and sesame, sunflower, and pumpkin seeds or their oils; lentils; and leafy green vegetables, plus lamb and grass fed beef.

Flaxseed oil, a highly nutritious oil rich in EFAs, is usually manufactured and distributed in opaque plastic containers. Unfortunately, it is difficult to find fresh, high-quality oils in the United States. When you do find them, they are more expensive than other oils—approximately $30 more per person per year—but considering the damage that improperly produced oil can cause, it is worth the investment (see appendix 1 for recommended sources).

WHEN NATURE CALLS, RESPOND

Paying attention "when nature calls" is essential to smoothly functioning bowels. Physiologically, human beings operate on a stimulus/response basis in regard to bodily functions. If you repeatedly ignore the urge to eliminate, you interfere with your body's ability to respond appropriately. Sooner or later, your body won't be able to function without artificial stimulation from medication, herbs, or water therapies such as enemas and colonics.

It is best to plan for proper elimination if you have a challenge in this area. Leave enough time in the morning after eating to allow the oral/anal reflex to work. When you chew food, you stimulate the inside of your mouth and a cascade of electrical and chemical events fires off, activating peristalsis within your gastrointestinal (GI) tract. Peristalsis is the muscular contraction that propels food down your digestive canal and feces out of your body. To respect your body's natural rhythms and to allow for easy elimination, it is helpful to be near a bathroom within an hour of eating.

EXERCISE THE WASTE
OUT OF YOUR BODY

Finally, if you want to have healthy, smoothly functioning bowels, it is important to engage in a regular exercise program, or at least to step up your activity level. All of the muscles in your body respond favorably to appropriate exercise, including the smooth muscle of your intestinal tract. The benefits of exercise have also been proven scientifically. A study involving people 65 and over showed that the group who exercised on a regular basis had more frequent and less difficult bowel movements than the group who did not.

In the 1970s before I knew about internal cleansing and all the steps you can take to support a healthy intestinal tract, my favorite remedy for constipation was to eat a raw carrot and go for a walk. That remedy was double-strength in that it included both the fiber and the exercise that stimulate bowel motility. Often one remedy alone will not work, but when combined with others, the force for healing multiplies. For more information about exercise, see chapter 15.

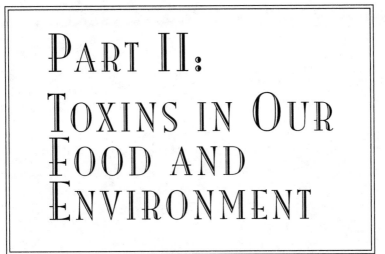

PART II:
TOXINS IN OUR FOOD AND ENVIRONMENT

CHAPTER 4

Toxins in Food

The Effect of Diet on Toxic Buildup in the Body

The Western diet has changed more in the last two centuries than at any previous time in human history. The changes have provided many conveniences, but they have also created new health threats. Chronic degenerative diseases build slowly and insidiously over a period of years until they gradually disrupt some part of your body. The most common killers are cardiovascular disease (of the heart and blood circulatory system); cancers; gastrointestinal diseases or disorders; arthritis; emphysema and other lung diseases; and diabetes and other endocrine system disorders. Medical science has proven that changes in our diet and lifestyle play an enormous role in the development of these diseases. Many of these diseases can be prevented by making informed changes in what you eat, what you think, how you move, and even in how you relate to your fellow human beings.

WHAT'S WRONG WITH THE AMERICAN DIET?

Since industrialization began over two hundred years ago, the Western diet has become increasingly rich in meats, poultry, saturated fats, refined foods, salt, sugar, and alcohol. Our overgenerous intake of animal fats has burdened our cardiovascular systems with cholesterol, our kidneys with protein, and our livers with animal hormones and drugs. Processed foods, which account for *more than half* of Americans' food intake, are loaded with salts; sugars; preservatives; and artificial, chemically altered ingredients. Every year, Americans spend more money on alcohol than our government does on the defense budget. We drink more soft drinks and coffee than ever before.

This change in diet is due to a new affluence in industrialized countries, to the availability of a wide variety of foods because of refrigeration and shipping, and to the overstimulation of our appetite centers by advertising campaigns of the food industry. The net result of these dietary changes since the early 1900s has been a 32 percent increase in fat consumption, a 50 percent increase in the consumption of sugar and other sweeteners, and a 43 percent increase in the consumption of carbohydrates. Increased consumption of fat (especially trans fats, which constitute up to 20 percent of the American diet) and refined carbohydrates leads to increased risk of heart disease, cancer, and diabetes, to name just a few diseases that have escalated with the modernization of the Western world.

Junk Food

Since the beginning of the twentieth century, the modern diet has become increasingly worse. Dr. Michael T. Murray, a naturopathic physician, provides the following statistics on the startling amount of junk food the average American consumes annually:

100 pounds of refined sugar
55 pounds of fats and oils
300 cans of soda pop
200 sticks of gum
18 pounds of candies
15 pounds of potato chips
63 dozen donuts
20 gallons of ice cream

Our national annual total for cola consumption is 100 billion ounces, and we spend $50 million on Twinkies. The food industry spends $8 billion annually on advertising these products. Close to 30 percent of Americans smoke cigarettes, and more than 7 percent are active alcoholics. On average, produce is shipped 1,800 miles before it reaches your table. To remain intact during shipping, the produce must be picked before it is fully ripe, and it sits in warehouses, in trucks, and on the grocery store shelves for days before you buy it. This means that the nutritive value is underdeveloped and depleted before the fruit or vegetable becomes food for your body.

Sugar

The average American consumes a shocking 100 pounds of sugar per year, which translates to approximately one-third of a pound per day. Excess sugar intake contributes to a wide variety of health problems, from tooth decay to heart disease, diabetes, hypoglycemia, obesity, and vaginal infections. Right from the start, babies' taste buds are perverted by the addition of simple sugars to baby formulas. I have seen mothers fill up bottles for their infants with artificially colored orange soda, and grandmothers put sugar in the water they serve to their grandchildren, beginning a lifetime addiction to sugar. In this chapter, you will learn why feeding sugar to infants sets them up to struggle with weight problems for the rest of their lives.

Salt

On average, Americans consume a whopping 8 pounds of salt per year. Have you ever read the ingredient label on a container of commercial table salt? It lists salt, sodium silicoaluminate, dextrose, potassium iodide, and sodium bicarbonate. What are all of these things doing in our salt? The addition of sodium silicoaluminate allows salt manufacturers to say that their salt is free-flowing. Putting some rice grains in your salt shaker can accomplish the same result without adding aluminum to your diet. Aluminum has been found in high concentrations in the brains of people with Alzheimer's disease. Dextrose (sugar) makes the salt taste sweet. Potassium iodide was added to salt after people in the Midwest, deprived of sources of ocean fish, developed goiter (enlargement of the thyroid gland). Sodium bicarbonate (baking soda) is an alkalizing agent, added to neutralize the acidity caused by the addition of the sweetness of the dextrose.

Salt comes from two places: the sea and dried-up ocean beds in the desert. If you want a pure form of salt, buy sea salt, rock salt, or kosher salt from your health food store or supermarket. None of these forms of salt has the additives of commercial table salt. However, they may be without the trace minerals you should be getting from natural salt sources. Look for *unrefined* sea salt, or you may end up with a product containing only sodium chloride.

Fats

The daily intake of calories from fat has more than tripled in the past two centuries, and the increase is mainly in the form of animal fat. Scientific data indicate that a diet rich in animal fat is strongly related to a high risk of heart disease and cancers of the colon, breast, and uterus. Heart disease is the leading cause of death in both Great Britain and the United States today, killing one out of every three people. Because large amounts of fat are difficult to digest, this excess may also lead to constipation, diarrhea, liver and gall bladder problems, menstrual and premenstrual difficulties, and skin disorders.

Low Fiber Intake

As you read in chapter 3, fiber is an important contributor to good bowel health. Fiber also plays an important role in preventing many degenerative diseases, primarily heart disease, diabetes, and colon- and hormone-related cancers. According to statistics, our daily intake of fiber is greatly reduced by the consumption of refined and processed foods. Fresh fruits and vegetables and whole grains, as opposed to refined rice or flour products, must be included in your daily diet to achieve a sufficient fiber supply for health and well-being. Some of you will not manage to ingest in your diet the 40 to 60 grams of fiber per day that is necessary for optimal health, so in chapter 7, I discuss supplements you can take to increase your daily fiber intake.

Overeating

With our poor diets and the lack of exercise in our daily schedules, it is easy to gain 10 to 20 pounds of excess weight. Weight gain may negatively impact your level of energy and self-esteem. It takes more energy to move more weight around, and if you are unhappy with your weight, you carry the additional psychological burden of disapproving of your body and yourself for not managing your weight better. Both of these factors contribute to depleting your energy reserves. As was discussed in chapter 1, negative self-talk leads to increased toxicity. Most likely the quality of the food and/or the proportion of protein, vegetable, and fat are not optimal, resulting in an increased toxic load. Experts in cardiovascular disease estimate that at least one-fourth of all heart disease problems can be attributed to overeating, which forces the heart and lungs to work harder than is healthy for them.

Body composition analysis with skin calipers, bio-impedance analysis, or immersion can measure the percentage of your weight that comes from fat, lean tissue (such as muscle, bone, and tendons), and water. Skin calipers measure body composition by measuring the depth of skin folds with a pinching device in places where fat usually accumulates (e.g., under the upper arm, around the waist). Bio-impedance analysis is a state-of-the-art tool that measures reactance and resistance to an extremely light electrical current that runs from two electrodes placed on one hand and foot on the dominant side of your body. The measurements are then entered into a computer that calculates percentages. Immersion in water is the last technique. After you are covered with grease and dressed in a bathing suit, you are immersed in a tub of water up to your neck. With this method, buoyancy and water displacement are measured to calculate body composition. Body composition analysis is a very helpful measurement to calculate during a cleansing program to ensure that you are not losing vital lean tissue.

Obesity is considered to be a measure of body fat equal to or greater than 30 percent of your total body weight. Obesity is the leading cause of high blood pressure, which in turn causes kidney damage, heart disease, and stroke. Hypertension (high blood pressure) is twice as common among overweight people as among lean people. Obese people have approximately four times the risk of developing diabetes and an increased risk of varicose veins, gout, respiratory diseases, gastrointestinal disorders, gall bladder and liver diseases, and arthritis compared with people of lower weight. All these conditions respond favorably to internal cleansing.

One of the most significant signs of risk for heart disease and diabetes is a waist-to-hip ratio greater than 0.95 for women and 0.75 for men. You can determine your ratio by measuring your waist (the smallest measurement between the bottom of your rib cage and above your navel) and your hips (the largest measurement around the widest part of your buttocks and upper thighs), then dividing your waist measurement by your hip measurement. For example, if you are a woman with a waist measurement of 28 and a hip measurement of 38, your ratio is 28 ÷ 38 = 0.74, well below the risk level. If your ratio is higher than the upper limit, it does not necessarily mean that you will manifest either disease, especially if you use your newfound knowledge to take action to improve your health.

To understand weight gain, we have to consider the nutritional value of food. The fundamental reason all creatures eat is to satisfy their nutritional requirements for living. Only human beings have developed food into a culinary art. When you eat sugar, alcohol, candy, or other refined carbohydrates (pasta, sourdough or white bread, rolls, cookies, cakes, and pastries), you drive up your need to eat more food, yet you feel satisfied only briefly because you are consuming "empty calories." Whenever you ingest a food or beverage other than pure water, you engage the metabolic (digestive) machinery in your body. The process of digestion requires energy and uses up key nutrients that are stored for this purpose. Refined foods do not contain the nutrients you need for their digestion, so you end up depleting your body's warehouse of stored nutrients. Because your basic needs are not met, you continue to be hungry, so you eat more than your body, mind, and heart need to thrive.

Caffeine

Twenty to 30 percent of American adults consume more than 500 milligrams of caffeine per day—twice the amount doctors consider a large "drug dose." An 8-ounce cup of coffee contains approximately 136 milligrams of caffeine. That means it takes four cups of coffee to total 544 milligrams of caffeine. Coffee, tea, cola beverages, and chocolate in all of its forms are the major sources of caffeine. Caffeine is also found in over-the-counter and prescription drugs. Studies performed in the past 10 years indicate that caffeine users have a 100 percent greater than average risk of heart attack.

There are several reasons to quit drinking coffee. Coffee is a narcotic beverage. The caffeine in your coffee belongs in the same alkaloid group of chemicals as morphine, cocaine, and strychnine. Drinking decaffeinated coffee is probably no better than drinking "hi-test" because of the large concentration of trichloroethylene, a potent liver carcinogen. Furthermore, growers use more pesticides on this crop than on any other. Some of the pesticides used on coffee plants over the past 20 years are aldrin, dieldrin, chlordane, and heptachlor. As if this toxic chemical application were not enough, the roasting process that brings out the aroma turns the oils in coffee into dangerous trans fats (discussed in chapter 3). Nitrosamines, poisons that naturally occur in coffee, are the same carcinogens that we avoid in bacon and other cured meats.

Ingesting caffeine places stress on your heart. Many people feel their heart race when they take their daily dose of caffeine. Because it drives your nervous system into a state of sympathetic alert—the state you attain when a wild animal is chasing you and you are running for your life— you become depleted in B-vitamins, especially B_1 (also called thiamin). (Symptoms of vitamin B_1 deficiency include fatigue, nervousness, general malaise, general aches and pains, and headaches.) Some people say they feel little of this "buzz" when they drink coffee. That is cause for real concern. If your adrenals do not react to the stimulation of caffeine, you could be headed for a physical breakdown due to adrenal exhaustion.

When you get into a state of sympathetic alert, your digestive system turns off because your blood is sent preferentially to your muscles, lungs, and heart. Any food in your digestive tract is subject to fermentation, putrefaction, and rancidity from sitting too long in an intestinal tract that is shut down. Instead of being nourished by your food, you become poisoned by the rotting products of incomplete digestion.

Coffee also interferes with your blood sugar metabolism. By stimulating a sympathetic response, it drives your blood sugar levels up and jolts your pancreas into action, flooding your system with insulin to normalize blood sugar levels. It puts your energy on a roller coaster ride all day long. People on this ride usually go from one caffeine high to the next, wearing out their glands and organs.

Because coffee is highly acidic, drinking it can lead to a deficiency of healthy bacteria in your intestines and make you subject to a host of health problems, including acne, constipation, diarrhea, recurring colds and flu, colitis, irritable bowel syndrome, and fibromyalgia.

If you still feel that you can't live without a caffeine buzz, try some green tea instead. Green tea is high in a substance called *catechin*. This flavonoid complex increases human resistance to certain types of cancers. You could also try jasmine tea or Earl Grey tea, both of which have lovely aromas and less caffeine than coffee.

Alcohol

When you drink an alcoholic beverage, the alcohol becomes a digestive priority and must be fully metabolized before anything else can be digested. The food you eat along with the alcohol you drink sits in your intestines waiting for its turn like a plane delayed on the runway. Depending on your ethnic background, your food may have a long wait. Native Americans, people of Irish descent, and Asians have a distinct disadvantage when it comes to digesting alcohol because of a genetic paucity of *alcohol dehydrogenase*, the enzyme that breaks down and neutralizes alcohol.

Alcohol consumption places a strain on the normal functions of your body. Alcohol disrupts our cells' ability to take in and use nutrients from food. It interferes with the absorption of numerous amino acids and increases the loss of certain vitamins in the urine, including pyridoxine and pantothenic acid (B-complex factors). It denies us the full benefit of what we eat. Heavy drinkers take in so many calories from alcohol that they tend to eat smaller quantities of nutritious food. To summarize, alcohol robs your body of nutrients essential for life.

Of course, we must remember the Taoist proverb, "Even moderation in moderation." There's nothing wrong with having an occasional drink unless it makes you sick or leads to self-destructive behavior.

TOXINS IN FOOD

Food, which is meant to nourish us, has become a significant source of internal pollution, both by design and by carelessness. Some 2,800 additives are intentionally added to what we eat. According to *Well Body, Well Earth,* the average American consumes about 14 pounds of additives a year. As many as 10,000 more additives find their way into food indirectly as it is grown, processed, packaged, and stored. These chemicals include hormones and antibiotics fed to animals, pesticides used on plants and crops, residues from substances used to clean equipment, molecules from plastic wrap, and lead from soldered cans. The U.S. Food and Drug Administration (FDA) does not require that these chemicals be listed on labels.

The most comprehensive food toxicity testing in the United States is the ongoing FDA Total Diet Survey. The findings regarding chlorinated pesticides thus far are alarming. DDE, a by-product of the pesticide DDT that can occur in the human body within 6 months of exposure to DDT, was found in

- 100 percent of samples of raisins, spinach, chili con carne, and beef
- 93 percent of samples of American processed cheese, hamburger, hot dogs, bologna, collards, chicken, turkey, and ice cream sandwiches
- 80 percent of samples of lamb chops, salami, canned spinach, meatloaf, and butter
- 81 percent of samples of cheddar cheese, pork sausage, white sauce, and creamed spinach

DDT has been banned for use in this country since 1972. Some of this contamination may be from other countries to whom we sell these chemicals.[1] According to Walter Crinion, a naturopathic physician, the most contaminated fruits and vegetables are strawberries, bell peppers, spinach, U.S. cherries, peaches, Mexican cantaloupe, celery, apples, apricots, green beans, Chilean grapes, and cucumbers.[2]

Pesticides in Baby Food

The Environmental Working Group (EWG) is a non-profit research organization based in Washington, D.C. In *Overexposed: Organophosphate Insecticides in Children's Food*, the EWG reports that in a study of eight non-organic baby foods produced by Gerber, Heinz, and Beech-Nut, the residues of 16 different pesticides were found, including probable human carcinogens, nervous system toxins that can harm the development of an infant's developing brain and nervous system, endocrine disrupters, and oral toxicity # 1 chemicals (No. 1 — the most toxic designation). The toxic levels found in these baby foods are based on the U.S. Environmental Protection Agency's current standards for pesticides in foods considered safe for adults, *not for infants*. We must remember that an infant weighs a fraction of what an adult human weighs, thereby increasing the poison concentrations five- to tenfold in a baby's body and amplifying their damaging effects.

According to the EWG report, Philip J. Landrigan, M.D., professor of Pediatrics and chair of the Department of Community and Preventive Medicine at Mt. Sinai Medical Center in New York City, has this to say: "Pesticides should not be allowed in baby food until they have been proven safe for infants." Dr. Landrigan chaired a 5-year study released by the National Academy of Sciences in 1993 that strongly recommended tougher safeguards to protect infants and children from pesticides.

Because industry and government have not taken the necessary steps to protect your infant or child from cancer, nervous system disease, and endocrine imbalance, it's up to you. You can protect your child by buying only organic foods, including organic baby food.

Chemically Altered Foods

Dr. George Goodheart, a chiropractor and founder of Applied Kinesiology, believes that males are being nutritionally castrated by the presence of trans fats, such as margarine, in our diets. To build healthy hormones, men (and women, for that matter) need biologically active fats and oils. These healthy fats and oils are converted by our digestive processes into testosterone, estrogen, and other hormones. Trans fats are not biologically active, however. They cannot be converted into our own hormones. They provide calories but no nutritional value. Trans fats are also found in chips, crackers, salad dressings, candies, cake frosting, and other processed foods and are called partially hydrogenated, hydrogenated, or fractionated on the product label.

Food companies take a perfectly good food—a polyunsaturated vegetable oil—and add hydrogen atoms to the double bonds in the long carbon chain attached to the hydroxyl portion of the fat. This alteration makes the oil solid and a more chemically stable compound with a longer shelf life. Unfortunately, the longer shelf life is dangerous to human life. In addition to the danger to our sex hormones, trans fats wreak havoc with our cardiovascular systems. Trans fats cause oxidative damage to the linings of our blood vessels. When this "nick" appears on the intima or inner lining of a blood vessel, a clot and plaque begin to form. If this newly formed "scab" dislodges from the artery wall, it may cause a blockage of a tiny artery upstream resulting in a heart attack or stroke.

Plastics in Food

In 1988, Drs. Ana Soto and Carlos Sonnenschein of Tufts University made an unexpected discovery while doing cancer research: "Phantom estrogen" coming from the plastic tubes in which they cultured their samples caused experimental colonies of breast cancer cells to multiply alarmingly. Eventually the researchers learned that the estrogenic substance was *p-nonylphenol*, one of the synthetic chemicals that manufacturers add to polystyrene and polyvinyl chloride (PVC) to make the materials more stable and less breakable. (P-nonylphenol is also used to synthesize nonoxynol-9 in birth control products such as contraceptive creams, foams, jellies, inserts, films, and condoms.)

Meanwhile, a Stanford University School of Medicine research team found another estrogenic mimic, *bisphenol-A*, in lab flasks and in such consumer products as giant jugs used for bottled drinking water. At the University of Granada, Spain, researchers Fatima and Nicolas Olea found bisphenol-A in the plastic coatings that manufacturers use to line metal cans. They also found an astonishingly high concentration of this estrogen mimic in such canned foods as corn, artichokes, and peas. In some instances the cans contained as much as 85 parts per billion bisphenol-A, 27 times the dose that the Stanford team found made breast cancer cells proliferate. The plastic linings are used to avoid possible contamination from tin and lead solder and to protect food from developing a metallic taste; they are found in 85 percent of food cans in the United States and 40 percent in Spain.

Non-stick cookware is another source of unexpected plastic exposure. The non-stick coating wears away, one fleck at a time, into your food. For the double-whammy toxic effect, your food comes more and more in contact with the aluminum surface underneath as the plastic surface erodes.

Here are some positive steps you can take to minimize the level of plastics in your food:

- Avoid microwaving food in plastic containers or with microwave plastic wrap. Reheat your food in ceramic or glass containers.
- Avoid allowing plastic juice and water containers to overheat (keep them out of hot cars and sunlight).

If the liquid becomes heated, throw it out. Or, buy juice and water in glass jars and bottles.

- Avoid eating food from cans. Instead, buy those foods frozen, dried, or in glass jars.
- Buy food fresh.
- Throw away your non-stick cookware. Cook your food in steel, glass, ceramic, or cast-iron cookware. Ask about the glaze on ceramics; some contain toxic metals such as lead.
- Avoid using contraceptive products that contain nonoxynol-9. Seek alternatives.

Bovine Somatotropic Hormone

Since 1994, most cow's milk sold in stores contains bovine somatotropic hormone (BSH). BSH is a synthetic hormone designed to increase a cow's milk production. Cows treated with BSH have a higher incidence of mastitis (a breast infection) and possibly cancers. This hormone passes from the cow's milk into those who drink it. The U.S. government does not require labeling of milk and milk products that carry this dangerous hormone. However, dairies that do not use BSH may state on their cartons that they never give their cows antibiotics or hormones. Cheeses imported from Europe do not contain BSH. To protect your health, ask your grocer or health food store manager to carry milk and milk products that do not contain this hormone. Or, better yet, drink goat's milk, or get the nutrients you normally derive from milk—primarily protein and calcium—from other food sources. Seaweed and mustard greens (and other leafy green vegetables) contain the highest concentrations of calcium in plant foods, though it's not as bioavailable.

READ INGREDIENT LABELS

Exercise caution when eating processed food. Read labels carefully, especially the lists of food ingredients and added chemicals. Ask an educated clerk in the store whether the list of additives includes helpful vitamin supplements with chemical names that make them sound like toxic additives. Your health-care practitioner may also be able to advise you in this regard.

Drugs in Food

Unfortunately, these toxins will not appear on the ingredient label. Antibiotics are being fed to the animals we eat for food. The antibiotics that beef and dairy cows, pigs, chicken, and fish have been treated with end up in our bodies when we eat their meat. Your only protection here is to eat organic foods, including organic animal and wild fish products. The WHO stated that the use of antibiotics in animals raised for food contributes to the problem of treatment-resistant bacteria that can be transmitted to humans through food.

On June 12, 2000, the World Health Organization (WHO) warned that increasingly drug-resistant infections in both rich and developing nations are threatening to make once treatable diseases incurable.[3] On June 13, 2000, the WHO issued guidelines aimed at cutting the use of antimicrobial treatments in animals raised for food. Half of the world's antibiotics are used on farms, sometimes to treat illness but mostly to make healthy animals grow bigger. According to the document, all such treatments should be subject to obligatory prescriptions, and national systems should be set up to monitor antimicrobial use and resistance.

The guidelines also say the use of antimicrobials to promote growth in animals should be ended or rapidly phased out if the drugs are also used for treating humans and they have not been evaluated for safety. "We're losing our window of opportunity," said WHO Infectious Diseases Chief Dr. David Heymann. "It's something we have to really address immediately or we're going to start losing our antibiotics." According to the WHO, drug-resistant *Salmonella* in European, Asian, and North American animals has caused diarrhea, blood poisoning, and death in humans. Gonorrhea was once easily curable with penicillin and tetracycline; "[t]oday, you can't touch it anywhere in the world with those drugs," Heymann said. Poor nations can't afford more expensive alternatives, and to make matters worse, untreated gonorrhea is fueling the spread of human immunodeficiency virus (HIV), the virus that causes AIDS.

Other alarming examples of drug resistance include the following:

- In Estonia, Latvia, and parts of Russia and China, more than 10 percent of people with tuberculosis have strains resistant to two powerful medicines. Overall, up to 2 percent of the world's 16 million people with tuberculosis have disease strains that are resistant to many drugs; this statistic is particularly frightening because tuberculosis is an airborne disease (i.e., it is spread through the air when people cough).
- Malaria, the mosquito-spread infection that kills a million people a year, is resistant to the top medication 80 percent of the time.

- Some 5,000 Americans may have suffered long-lasting food poisoning in 1998 from drug-resistant germs in chicken.
- The Center for Disease Control says that 88,000 Americans a year die from infections they catch in the hospital, and many of these infections are resistant to at least one antibiotic, complicating treatment attempts.

The FDA has debated stricter rules for several years (Europe has already banned several such drugs) but is under industry pressure not to tighten animal drug restrictions.[4]

Mother's Milk

The substances a nursing mother puts in her body including foods and drugs are fed to her baby through her breast milk. It is common for a nursing mother to adapt her eating regimen to prevent upset in her infant's digestive tract. What has not been strongly considered in the past is the effect of prescription drugs on the nursing baby.

L. H. Chaudron and J. W. Jefferson from the William S. Middleton Memorial Veterans Affairs Hospital and the University of Wisconsin Medical School studied the effects of the use of mood-stabilizer drugs (such as antidepressants) during breastfeeding by reviewing medical databases: "The search revealed 11 cases of lithium use during breastfeeding, 8 of which reported infant serum levels. Two cases reported symptoms consistent with lithium toxicity in the infants. Thirty-nine cases of valporate use during breastfeeding were found, 8 of which reported infant serum levels. There was

1 report of thrombocytopenia and anemia in an infant. Fifteen cases of carbamazepine use during breastfeeding were found, 10 of which reported infant serum levels. Two infants experienced hepatic (liver) dysfunction."[5] What these investigators found is that the antidepressant drugs used by the mother showed up in her infant's blood. In two cases, the drugs caused damage to the babies' livers; another had anemia and a deficiency of the cells that help blood to clot to stop bleeding. Two other infants suffered with lithium toxicity as a result of their mothers' prescription drug intake. Nursing mothers may wish to discuss alternatives to mood altering drugs, such as exercise, with their healthcare practitioner. Studies show that exercise alone can be as effective in controlling even severe depression as prescription medications but without any damage to the nursing infant.

CHAPTER 5

HOUSEHOLD AND OTHER PERSONAL TOXINS

MINIMIZING RISKS INSIDE THE HOME

Toxic vapors are released from materials found in your home and office through a phenomenon known as "out-gassing": Emissions include formaldehyde from particle-board furniture; volatile organic compounds (VOCs) from stains, varnishes, and paint; resins from adhesives that hold furniture and built-in units together; and numerous compounds from plastic household and office items, cleaning products, synthetic carpets, drapes, and upholstery. Wood furniture and furnaces, gas ranges, and wood stoves also emit natural vapors.

Indoor air pollution is linked to many health concerns, including asthma. A National Academy of Sciences (NAS) press release on January 19, 2000, was titled, "Study Finds Strong Evidence that Exposure to Some Indoor Substances Can Lead To or Worsen Asthma." According to the NAS, sources of common allergens include:

- dust mites and cockroaches
- fungi and mold
- dander, hair, and saliva from domestic pets and other animals
- viruses and bacteria
- spores and materials from houseplants
- secondhand smoke
- pesticides
- cleaning and building materials[1]

Ways to "Clear the Air"

A brochure from the Florida Foliage Association recommends placing approximately 15 plants in an 1,800-square-foot house to combat indoor air pollution. Five plants are listed in their brochure as especially helpful:

- Chinese evergreen *(Aglaonema* "Silver Queen")
- spider plant *(Chlorophytum comosum* "Vittatum")
- peace lily *(Spathiphyllum* species)
- golden pothos *(Epipremnum aureum)*
- weeping fig *(Ficus benjamina)*

Indoor plants are particularly effective in filtering three chemicals from the air that are responsible for many health problems: benzene, formaldehyde, and trichloroethylene (TCE).

Benzene is a common solvent and is present in gasoline, inks, oils, paints, plastic, rubber, detergents, pharmaceuticals, and dyes. It causes symptoms such as: headaches, loss of appetite, drowsiness, nervousness, psychological disturbances, and diseases of the blood system including anemia and bone marrow disease. Evidence also links benzene to cancer, leukemia, liver and kidney damage, paralysis, and unconsciousness. (Benzene is also found in canned soda.)

Formaldehyde irritates the mucous membranes of your eyes and upper respiratory system. Recent research also suggests that it may cause a rare form of throat cancer in long-term occupants of mobile homes. I have learned that Boston ferns are happy to soak up formaldehyde that outgasses from particleboard, pressed wood furniture, and foam insulation in your home or office. Consumer paper products, including grocery bags, waxed paper, facial tissue, and paper towels, are also treated with formaldehyde resins.

TCE is used in metal degreasers, dry-cleaning agents, inks, paints, lacquers, varnishes, and adhesives. The National Cancer Institute (NCI) considers TCE a potent liver carcinogen. I was informed by one of my patients that if you have seventeen spider plants in your home, then your air will be clean. Try what she does: Systematically cultivate the "baby spiders" from the first plant until you reach the recommended quota.

As a part of the photosynthesis process, plants take in carbon dioxide along with airborne toxins and turn them into oxygen for us to breathe. Plants also help clean the air of auto and industrial exhaust, thereby making the world a healthier place for all of us to live. These are only a few reasons why it is so very important for us to protect the plant population on our planet.

You might consider purchasing an air cleaner for your home. They come in a variety of styles; some produce ozone to kill mold, some produce negative ions to precipitate particulate pollutants, and some move air through a carbon (to

remove gasses) or a HEPA (high-efficiency particulate ac-
cumulator) filter. Combination air filters with a charcoal and
a central HEPA filter are probably the most useful. In my
home, I use a combination ultraviolet, ion, and air filter. In
my office, we use a combination filter when necessary (such
as when mold or pollution levels are high or when patients
come in wearing scented products on their hair or body).
Check appendix 1 and *Consumer Reports* for valuable information about air filtration.

A few more ways to keep your home healthy include
the following:

- Don't smoke inside the house or around your children, elderly people, or people who are sick.
- Invest in a "clean air" vacuum cleaner that prevents
  dust from venting through the vacuum bag and
  back into your home.
- Avoid using insecticides or pesticides in and around
  your home.
- Use the safe cleaning products described later in
  this chapter.

Household Cleaning Products: Safer Alternatives

You can replace all of the toxic cleaners lurking under your
sinks (be sure to dispose of these toxic items safely) with
just a few simple solutions of baking soda, white vinegar,
olive oil, borax, and lemon juice. For safer cleaning in the
home, use these "recipes for healthy household cleaners,"
adapted from *Creative Reuse Extravaganza,* by Cynthia Ashley
and Sylvia Valazques.

- **All-purpose cleaner**—Pour undiluted white vinegar into a spray bottle. You will be amazed at what it will clean, and it will not harm surfaces.
- **Carpet freshener**—Sprinkle baking soda over the carpet. Let it sit for several hours to absorb unwanted odors, then vacuum it.
- **Floor and furniture polish**—Mix one part lemon juice (reconstituted is just fine; if you use fresh lemons, strain out the pulp and seeds) and two parts olive oil in a jar or bottle; shake well. Pour a small amount of the mixture onto furniture or the floor, and rub well with a rag.
- **Laundry brightener**—Add one-half cup of white vinegar, baking soda, or borax to each load of washing to brighten dingy, dirty clothes without harming them.
- **Moth repellent**—Place a handful of cedar chips and/or lavender flowers in a small square of netting or other sheer material, such as old nylons or pantyhose, to make a sachet. Tie it closed with wire or ribbon and hang in your closet or place in drawers to keep moths away.
- **Toilet bowl cleaner**—Sprinkle about ½ cup of baking soda or borax into the toilet bowl. Add a small amount of white vinegar. Scrub with a toilet brush.
- **Window cleaner**—Mix one part white vinegar with one part water in a spray bottle; shake well. If the smell of vinegar is too strong, mix one part vinegar and two parts water. Even diluted, the mixture is still an effective window cleaner.

Water Filtration Systems

If you are concerned about safe drinking water, there is hope in point-of-use filtration systems that use a water filter at the kitchen faucet (see chapter 6 for more on dirty drinking water). Your greatest exposure to chlorine, however, is not from drinking but from taking showers. Soaking in a bathtub also exposes you to significant chlorine fumes. If you like taking baths and want to protect yourself from the chlorine in the bathwater, you can do what friends of mine do. They heat up filtered water on the stove and transport the heated water into their tub in big pots. If you don't want to work that hard, consider filling your tub with water flowing through a shower head filter, whole-house filtration, or a point-of-use filter in the bathroom. Fortunately, several high-quality water purification systems are on the market.

Various types of water filtration and purification systems are available. Sediment filters remove dirt, rust, and silt. Carbon block filters improve the taste and odor of water by removing chlorine and chlorine by-products. Ozone treatments will remove chlorine also. Ultraviolet light kills bacteria. Reverse osmosis (RO) membranes block heavy metals such as mercury, lead, fluorine, cadmium, and arsenic as well as inorganic mineral salts. They enable carbon filters to do a better job and should be used only with a carbon block as a first-stage filter because they are not chlorine resistant. A storage tank is required with an RO membrane filter. A carbon post-RO filter removes residual taste, odors, and organic minerals.

When considering a water filtration unit for your home, ask yourself five questions:

1. Does this system remove all or most of the toxic compounds that could be harmful to human health?
2. Is it cost-effective?
3. Is it easy to install and maintain?
4. Is it friendly to the environment?
5. Does the filtered water taste good?

According to Dr. Jeffrey Bland, a nutritional bio-chemist, the best water purification systems include pre- and post-compressed charcoal filters with an RO membrane in between the two charcoal filters. During the water filtration process, water first goes into a pre-charcoal filter, then through the RO membrane, and finally through the post-charcoal filter. These filtration units must be placed below the sink and usually are installed by a plumber. Because they contain more working parts than other types of water filters, they are more costly to purchase and maintain, but they are often available at warehouse clubs. They also use approximately 1 gallon of water for every gallon that they purify. The charcoal filters must be replaced every 6 months, adding to the solid waste in our landfills.

You may need to add additional stages to an under-the-counter water filter depending on the harmful solvents in your water supply. In addition, if you buy a water filter with replacement cartridges, make sure that replacement cartridges are readily available, because the effectiveness of a water filter depends on regular maintenance.

A word of warning about the widely available hand-held pitcher-type water filters, which consist of only granular carbon particles: These filters may actually increase your exposure to disease-producing microorganisms. In time, the tap water no longer comes in contact with the charcoal granules because channels are formed as the water repeatedly runs through the unit. Eventually, residue from previously filtered water collects on these channels and acts as a breeding ground for harmful microorganisms.

HOUSEHOLD PESTICIDES

Did you ever consider that mowing your lawn could be hazardous to your health? An article in the October 14, 1991, *Wall Street Journal* reported the case of Tom Latimer, a vigorous, athletic man with a bright future as a petroleum engineer. One Saturday morning after an hour of cutting the grass, picking up clippings, and edging the walkways around his home, he felt dizzy and nauseated. His nose was running, his chest was tight, and he had a pounding headache. Ten days later, he was getting sicker. He suffered with constant head pain, and his eyes began to jerk uncontrollably. Within months, he developed testicular cancer. Six years and twenty doctors later, Latimer accepted the diagnosis that he had been poisoned by an organophosphate pesticide. Earlier that fateful summer when he first experienced symptoms, he had sprayed an organophosphate pesticide on some anthills and insect nests in his yard.

Normally, the liver can detoxify small amounts of a pesticide in 1 or 2 days, but Latimer had a complicating factor: He was taking Tagamet, which is generally prescribed to control excessive stomach acid. Alfredo Sadun, Ph.D., a professor of neurosurgery and ophthalmology at the University of Southern California, says that taking a medication such as Tagamet "can make a person 100 to 1,000 times more sensitive to organophosphate poisoning." Tagamet and non-steroidal anti-inflammatory drugs (NSAIDs) such as Aleve, Motrin, Tylenol, and aspirin interfere with the cytochrome P450 pathway—the liver's first phase of detoxification. Latimer and his wife had both worked in the yard in bare arms and shorts, digging around flowerbeds and shrubbery that had been treated with the pesticide. His wife wasn't taking Tagamet, and she didn't get sick.

Tom Latimer can no longer ride a bike. He has difficulty walking. At night, to combat brain seizures and nightmares, he takes an anti-epileptic medicine. His sleep is disturbed, and annual laser surgery has to be performed to remove viral growths on his vocal cords due to suppression of his immune system caused by xenobiotic (man-made chemical) exposure. His personal life and professional life have been irreversibly damaged. With Latimer's natural defenses compromised by the combination of Tagamet and pesticides, the poison carried out a potent and ongoing attack on his nervous system.

A growing body of research indicates that many Americans may be vulnerable to chronic, low-level exposure to pesticides, which can produce severe abdominal pain, headaches, nausea, and other effects. Recent estimates suggest that each year there are three million severe pesticide poisonings (including accidents such as spills, unprotected agriculture application, and factory explosions) and 220,000 deaths worldwide. In the United States, pesticide-related illnesses are estimated to occur between 150,000 and 300,000 times a year. Over time, the risks from exposure vary depending on a number of factors such as individual sensitivity levels and immune suppression, but these risks may include cancer; birth defects; and damage to the liver, kidneys, and nervous system.

In an October 1994 *Medical Hypothesis* article titled "Neurasthenic Fatigue, Chemical Sensitivity, and GABA Receptor Toxins," F. M. Corrigan and S. MacDonald reported that low levels of insecticides and polychlorinated biphenyls (PCBs) found in our environment and the body fat of humans may be the cause of chronic fatigue syndromes, including multiple chemical sensitivities in susceptible individuals. Other symptoms and disorders caused by exposure to pesticides and PCBs include throat irritation and dryness, bouts of profuse sweating, headaches, muscle pains, weakness, concentration difficulties, joint pains, palpitations, chest pain and tightness, reduced tolerance for alcohol, dizziness, elevated Epstein-Barr titer, cognitive dysfunction, back pain, swollen glands, hypersensitivity to light, decreased appetite, sleepiness, anxiety, atrial fibrillation, irritability, indecisiveness, depression, personality change, and flu-like symptoms. Elevated Epstein-Barr titer is closely associated with chronic fatigue immunodeficiency syndrome (CFIDS).

The problem with public warnings about such risks is that neither the U.S. Food and Drug Administration (FDA) nor the U.S. Environmental Protection Agency (EPA) test for toxicity from combined chemicals, even those commonly used together. Testing for the effects of combinations of medications and chemicals is far beyond their reach.

In the June 1996 issue of *Science* magazine, a group of researchers from Tulane University reported on a preliminary investigation into the effect of combined pesticides that by themselves have little effect on the activity of estrogen. When combined, however, their stimulation of estrogen receptors and activity was increased. A surplus of estrogen has been linked to breast cancer and malformation of male sex organs. John A. McLachlan, principal investigator, reported, "If you test them individually, you could conclude that they were nonestrogenic, almost inconsequential. But when we put them in combination, their potency jumped up 500- to 1000-fold."

In *Our Stolen Future*, authors Theo Colborn, Dianne Dumanovski, and John Peterson Myers stated, "Hormonally active synthetic chemicals are thugs on the biological information highway that sabotage vital communication. They mug the messengers or impersonate them. They jam signals. They scramble messages. They sow misinformation. They wreak all manner of havoc." And this havoc seems to spread across generations.

Because PCBs show up in our water supplies and the fish that swim in them, Helen Daly and a team of researchers at State University of New York at Oswego fed rats a diet that included salmon from nearby Lake Ontario in 1992. They found behavioral problems; when confronted with mildly negative situations, the fish-fed rats became "hyperreactive," reported Daly. Not only were the rat pups affected, but the mother's behavior was also abnormal. Even more startling was the finding that the mother rat's grandchildren overreacted as well. This finding is very significant. Even though the second- and third-generation rats were not exposed to PCBs, they suffered damage as a consequence of the first-generation female's exposure. (The same results have been seen with zinc deficiency. The offspring for two generations show signs that include a weakened immune system. Even receiving sufficient quantities of zinc cannot make up for their grandmother's zinc deficiency. Adult humans

need from 40 to 80 milligrams of zinc in their diet per day.)
Daly has shown that this cross-generational effect is not gender biased, at least in rats. And tragically, in May 1995, the
Oswego team announced that they had found similar behavioral effects in human children.

Pesticides and other *xenobiotics* (chemical compounds
that are foreign to a living organism) can affect the sex hormones in your body. Depending on the chemical, they may
stimulate hormone production, or they may lower hormone
levels by accelerating their breakdown and elimination,
thereby leaving your body short of not only estrogen but of
testosterone and other hormones as well. Hormones are produced by endocrine glands, including the thyroid, thymus,
pancreas, adrenal glands, ovaries, and testicles. Hormones
regulate a multitude of functions, including brain development, energy level, immune system function, sugar metabolism, stress response, bone strength, sex drive, sexual
characteristics, and fertility. The adrenal glands, which produce stress hormones, are affected by xenobiotic compounds
more than any other organ, followed by the thyroid gland.

Many of us know about the temperature-regulating
effects of the thyroid gland and how the activity of the thyroid determines our basal and resting metabolic rates, which
in turn influence your weight. But the thyroid is also needed
in the development of the brain. Research has shown that
thyroid hormones stimulate the production and placement of
nerve cells within the brain. Pesticides such as PCBs and
dioxins mimic or block this hormone action. Problems resulting from interference with natural hormones range from
mental retardation to behavioral disorders such as hyperactivity and learning disabilities such as attention deficit hyperactivity disorder (ADHD).

Cross-Generational Toxicity

A severe example of pesticide poisoning is seen in the children born to Taiwanese women who ate cooking oil that was accidentally contaminated[2] with high levels of PCBs and furans. Furans are flammable liquids made synthetically or from pine oil. They have toxic effects similar to dioxins, of which the most infamous is Agent Orange, used in the Vietnam War. Dioxin has earned its reputation as the most dangerous synthetic chemical as a result of the damage suffered by soldiers exposed to Agent Orange (for more information about this toxic agent of war, see chapter 6).

The children of the Taiwanese women exposed to PCBs and furans suffered a range of health defects, including the sexual organ effects that we have become familiar with from investigation of other hormone-stimulating xenobiotics. For instance, boys exposed to PCBs and furans had significantly shorter penises than boys of the same age not exposed. In general, the children showed permanent impairment in their motor and coordination skills and mental abilities. Behavioral problems including hyperactivity made it difficult for them to concentrate and to learn.

Children whose mothers ate Lake Michigan fish during their pregnancies showed similar effects.[3] The women ate the fish only twice per month in the 6 years prior to pregnancy, and some had none while pregnant. The more fish the mother ate, the smaller her baby's head, which suggests decreased brain size and intelligence. The babies also had a lower birth weight than did the group of women who had consumed no fish. They exhibited weak reflexes and more jerky movements. At 7 months, they showed impaired cognitive function, which includes all aspects of perceiving, thinking, and remembering. And at 4 years of age, the children of women with the highest PCB levels had lower scores in verbal and memory tests. In both groups of children—the Taiwanese and the Lake Michigan—the chemicals the pregnant mothers were exposed to interfered with the babies' thyroid's ability to optimally organize their brains while they were developing in the womb.

PCBs: A Toxic Legacy

On May 22, 2000, the Chicago Associated Press reported that a federal study shows that more than 20 years after the manufacture of PCBs was banned, the cancer-causing toxins are still entering Lake Michigan from sources on land. The toxins may be coming from old electrical transformers, dumps that were not capped properly, sludge beds, and disposal sites for PCB-laced sediment dredged from rivers and shipping canals, said Tom Holsen, an environmental engineering professor at Clarkson University in New York, who is leading the PCB study in Chicago. PCBs have been linked to cancer and birth defects. The chemical was widely used as a coolant in electrical transformers during the 1960s and 1970s, to control dust on roads, as a wood preservative, and in paints.

Since 1995, tests have also found high levels of PCBs near Baltimore, Maryland, Detroit, Michigan, and in England. Many government officials and advocacy groups support dredging contaminated sediment from lakes and rivers. Industry has resisted, claiming it is too expensive and has favored covering polluted sediment with clean fill (such as clay) to limit exposure, said Glenn Warren of the EPA's Great Lakes National Program Office in Chicago. Meanwhile, we continue to be exposed.

Pesticides and Cancer

The following common household pesticides have a positive association between exposure and brain cancer:

- No-Pest strips
- termite treatment
- Kwell shampoo (lindane)
- flea collars for pets
- diazinon use in the garden or orchard
- herbicides in the yard
- home pesticide bombs[4]

Other studies of children and toxic exposure have found 2,4-D (a common weed killer, which was added to 2,4,5-T to form Agent Orange) use around the home was associated with soft-tissue sarcomas.[5] The use of No-Pest strips and household and garden pesticides was associated with leukemia and household insecticide use with non-lymphocytic leukemia.[6]

Adults are affected, too. The use of chlorophenoxy acid herbicides such as 2,4-D has been strongly associated with increased incidence of lung cancer, stomach cancer, leukemia, Hodgkin's lymphoma, non-Hodgkin's lymphoma, and soft-tissue sarcomas. 2,4-D is commonly used by cities and states as a spray on roadways and rights-of-way to inhibit weed growth. It can be purchased at home stores for home lawn care and is often applied by chemical lawn companies.[7] Don't use these poisons. There are other options.

Alternatives to Toxic Pesticides

Use natural pest control. Ask your local organic farmers, contact your local library, or check with your local nursery about alternatives to dangerous chemical pesticides. I use McKenzie Rock Flour and compost from kitchen plant waste to keep my plants healthy (see appendix 1 for more information). Like humans, if plants are fed the proper nutrients, they will have greater resistance to disease.

To rid your home of such pests as ants and cockroaches, try diatomaceous earth. Diatomaceous earth is a natural pesticide that works by mechanical action instead of chemical action. This avoids the problem of pests that adapt by mutating into pesticide-resistant future generations, as is the case with chemical pesticides. Diatomaceous earth also can be used to de-worm your animals—especially horses.

Nematodes can be used to deal with termite infestation; the nematode parasitizes and kills termites. (Note that nematode treatment cannot be applied in areas where termite sprays have been previously used.) Other less toxic methods for dealing with termites include electricity, heat treatment, and freezing. You can also find safe alternatives to pesticides in the Gardens Alive! catalog and from the Bio-Integral Resource Center (BIRC) organization in Berkeley (see appendix 1).

MERCURY AMALGAM FILLINGS

Modern dentists can correct the effects of bad diet and improper oral hygiene by drilling and filling cavities, performing root canals, and providing caps and bridges. But there appear to be risks from dental procedures. Many cutting-edge dentists are seeing the ill effects of "silver" fillings (which contain mercury and other metal and nonmetal compounds), mercury amalgam fillings, and metal posts that are secured into the jaw in root canals.

Mercury amalgam fillings may be a significant factor contributing to bad health. Dr. Jeffrey Bland recommends that anyone with adult acne, neurological problems, or autoimmune disorders consider working with a dentist who specializes in removing mercury amalgam fillings and replacing them with composite fillings. Other symptoms of mercury toxicity, according to Dr. Michael Lebowitz, a chiropractor who specializes in helping the chronically ill, are depression, memory loss, food sensitivities, and "weird neuropathies." Neuropathies—functional disturbances or pathological changes in the peripheral nervous system—usually manifest as unusual sensations in the arms and legs, such as numbness and tingling.

In Europe, the problem of amalgam use is being taken seriously in professional circles. Countries such as Sweden and Austria have restricted or eliminated the use of amalgam fillings, and Germany's leading supplier of amalgam is getting out of the market. For the sake of patients, dentists, and dental assistants, mercury amalgam will be replaced by other materials before too long.

In the United States in 1994, approximately 6 percent of dentists recognized the danger of mercury amalgam fillings. Because it is a recently recognized danger, your dentist may not know much about the topic. The American Dental Association's stance is that no dangers are associated with this material, and they make no moves to restrict its use.

Unfortunately, the time of greatest exposure to mercury from fillings is both during filling and removal. If you are going to have your fillings removed and replaced with composite material, I recommend that you work with a dentist who takes precautions against mercury exposure (for more information on mercury fillings, see appendix 1).

Some people have complete immune system breakdowns after having their fillings taken out. Here are three precautions you should take to minimize your risk:

1. Make sure your whole mouth is covered with a rubber dam during removal.
2. Wear a mask or get oxygen during the procedure.
3. Have a shot of DMPS or oral DMSA (chelating agents that take mercury out of your body) immediately after removal.

TOXIC DRUG REACTIONS

On April 30, 2000, the London *Sunday Times* detailed the history of several families who have experienced complications related to the measles mumps rubella (MMR) vaccine. One family involved triplets and a single mother; all three of the triplets have been profoundly affected, according to the mother. Another family related the story of a child who was vaccinated shortly before Christmas 1995. Christmas Eve videotapes show a happy playful child, and Christmas Day videotapes show a damaged child. In 1998 Andrew Wakefield published an article in *Lancet* linking autism and gastrointestinal changes with the MMR vaccine. The 12 children studied lost previously acquired skills including language or the ability to talk along with abdominal pain and diarrhea.[8] Japan has outlawed the MMR vaccine; France and Japan offer immunization for mumps, measles, and rubella as individual shots (this comes from the London *Sunday Times* April 30, 2000). In a private conversation recently with Dr. Jeffrey Bland, nutritional biochemist, noted international lecturer, and author of several books on health, he stated that it would be more prudent to immunize children against infectious diseases between 2 to 4 years of age when their immune systems have had the ability to mature to some degree.

EVERYDAY TOXINS

Even the current use of antibacterial or antimicrobial soaps is dangerous. Hexachlorophene (HCP) added to soap to kill germs causes damage to myelin, the protective sheath that surrounds nerves. (People with multiple sclerosis show evidence of myelin damage.) HCP is readily absorbed through intact skin and mucous membranes. Other negative health effects attributed to HCP are blurred vision and muscular weakness, progressing to paralysis.[9]

2,4-Diaminoanisole sulfate, a common ingredient in hair dye, caused thyroid cancer when fed to rats at high doses.[10]

Sources of toxins present themselves in many ways and from many fronts. To effectively reduce your toxic load, you must first be able to recognize where they came from and then minimize their impact on your life. Because you cannot completely escape toxic exposure, cleansing programs are essential to improve your health. Read parts III and IV of this book for help finding your way more safely through our polluted world.

CHAPTER 6

ENVIRONMENTAL TOXINS

It is virtually impossible to escape toxic substances. Air is everywhere. Water evaporates into the atmosphere, circulates, and rains down onto the Earth's surface, where it drains into streams, rivers, and oceans. Strong air and water currents carry pollution to the farthest reaches of the north and south poles.

HOW ENVIRONMENTAL TOXINS MOVE UP THE FOOD CHAIN

Humans eat at the top of the food chain, which means eating other animals, birds, and fish, as opposed to eating plants and algae exclusively. Like humans, plants and animals store toxins in their fatty parts. Toxins move up the food chain from plants, bugs, and algae to small fish and mammals, which are then eaten by large fish and mammals, which are consumed by humans. Toxins are also passed on to newborns through breast milk. At each level of the food chain, toxins become more concentrated.

The May 13, 1996, *Los Angeles Times* published an article about the effect of pollution on the human immune system. The Inuit people of Arctic Canada, although far from industrialization, are believed to be the most highly contaminated humans on Earth. The world's pollution is carried to them on northbound air and ocean currents and is present in the native foods that they eat. The Inuit eat mostly fish and marine mammals, whose bodies carry high concentrations of fat to protect them from frigid arctic waters and from starvation when food is scarce. Because of this, the bulk of the Inuit diet includes very concentrated levels of toxins.

Perhaps the most tragic part of the story is that the toxins accumulated in the bodies of fish and marine mammals are even more concentrated in breast milk. The *Los Angeles Times* reported that Inuit babies have low B- and T-cell counts (produced by the body's cells and thymus gland, respectively, in response to invading microorganisms) from immune system suppression caused by feeding on their mothers' breast milk, which has high concentrations of PCBs (polychlorinated biphenyls) and DDT. PCBs are used to insulate electrical transformers far from Broughton Island, where the Inuit live, and DDT is used thousands of miles away from their Canadian Arctic region. Yet these dangerous chemicals reach the Inuit and are then passed on to their children. Inuit children take in seven times more PCBs than the typical infant in southern Canada or the United States. A 1995 study found various abnormalities in the immune systems of these children; for example, their bodies do not produce the necessary antibodies when vaccinated for smallpox, measles, polio, and other diseases. The increased rate of infection also leads to loss of hearing in one out of four children.

POLLUTION AND IMMUNOSUPPRESSION

Pollution, however, is not restricted to the north pole. Children who live near tanning factories in the southern part of the United States have a higher rate of leukemia than the general population. Many of the survivors of the radiation explosion at Chernobyl in the former Soviet Union need bone marrow transplants to produce red blood cells just to stay alive. In the *Los Angeles Times* article cited previously, Steve Hollanday, an immunotoxicologist at Virginia-Maryland Regional College of Veterinary Medicine, stated, "We're probably all—and I mean the whole doggone planet—immunosuppressed."

Immunosuppression is a condition in which the body does not have the strength and resilience to fight off bacteria, viruses, and parasites. As a result, cells that have been damaged by pollution and drugs will not be recognized and destroyed. If damaged cells are not destroyed, they may multiply and divide, reproducing themselves as mutated cells, which may in turn develop into cancer.

FALLING SPERM COUNTS

Men should pay particular attention to the following information about chemical effects that decrease male potency and cause malformation of male sex organs. Sperm counts are dropping for all species across the planet. To count sperm, we measure millions of sperm per milliliter of semen.

In the past five decades, the count has been dropping by approximately one million sperm per milliliter each year. Since 1938, with the rise of industrialization, human male sperm count has dropped by half. To have the pool from which future generations will emerge cut in half in less than a century is a shocking threat to the future of humanity. Studies from Scotland, Belgium, and France in the early 1990s showed an inverse correlation between the year of birth and the health of a man's sperm. Men born in 1945 and measured in 1975 averaged 102 million sperm per milliliter of semen. Men born in 1962 and measured in 1992 averaged 51 million. If this trend continues, by 2005, a thirty-year-old man would have a sperm count equaling just 25 percent of that of the average male born in 1925. If we don't change our lifestyle, will men be producing any sperm by 2042?

The quantity of sperm is not the only factor we need to consider. As we move forward in time, more sperm are deformed and miss their target because they don't swim right; the incidence of testicular cancer has jumped sharply, and genital abnormalities such as undescended testicles and shortened urinary tracts are on the rise. This is a problem, *but* there is a way out of the dilemma: cleansing, and lifestyle changes.

One way to decrease exposure to pollutants and their negative effects on your health and sperm count is to eat organic fruit and vegetables. A Danish study that compared farmers to airline workers was reported in the June 30, 1996, issue of the *San Francisco Examiner*. Each group was analyzed for their sperm count. The group of organic farmers, at least one-quarter of whose diet was pesticide-free produce, had sperm counts 43 percent higher than those of the airline workers.

Pesticides are designed to kill living things. And much to the distress of our health and fertility as a species, our bodies mistake these xenobiotic compounds for our own estrogens. Estrogen is the hormone that is responsible for creating female characteristics and is present in highest concentrations in women; testosterone is the hormone responsible for male sexual and behavioral characteristics and is present in highest concentrations in men. Men exposed to increasing amounts of estrogenic compounds are being feminized by a lowered ratio of testosterone to estrogen, possibly because receptor sites for male hormones are blocked by estrogenic substances.

The *San Francisco Examiner* article also mentioned other factors that may be involved in decreasing sperm counts. These factors correspond to greater exposure to harmful chemicals through city living versus country living and eating processed versus whole foods.

DIRTY WATER

Often you hear news reports about a new contamination problem in the water supplies throughout the United States. According to the U.S. Environmental Protection Agency (EPA), there are nearly 200,000 active surface impoundments (ground-level collection sites for toxic chemicals) in the United States, of which about 26,000 are unlined and may be leaking a wide variety of toxic chemicals into underground water supplies (see Figure 6.1). John Skinner, a director of the EPA's Office of Solid Waste Programs, reported in a congressional hearing that 95 percent of all operating surface impoundments are located within one-quarter of a

Toxic chemicals that are dumped are dissolved by rains and percolate into the ground. Plumes are then formed in ground water that bring these chemicals up in wells that tap the water sources. Septic tanks, sewers, toxic waste dumps, waste pits, and disposal wells all send toxic chemicals into the streams and fresh water wells.

Figure 6.1   Groundwater Contamination   (Reprinted by permission of Jon Goodchild from *Well Body, Well Earth.*)

mile of drinking water supplies. Once groundwater has become contaminated, it is almost impossible to purify.

Beginning on December 1, 1996, the *San Francisco Examiner* published a three-part series on water quality, concluding, "The nation's drinking water is at risk." Water pipes are aging, population is booming, and germs in our water are becoming more resistant to the chemicals traditionally used to kill them. In 1993, 403,000 people in Milwaukee got sick and 104 died from contamination by the microbe *Cryptosporidium*. The same year, residents of New York City and Washington, D.C., were warned to boil their water before drinking it because it contained pathogenic *E. coli* (fecal bacteria). Since then, at least 850 other community water systems have been ordered to boil their water. In 1995, the U.S. Centers for Disease Control and Prevention (CDC) advised people with weakened immune systems, such as those with AIDS or who have undergone chemotherapy or organ transplants, to boil water, use filters, or drink certain bottled waters. (For more information, contact the CDC in Atlanta, Georgia, at 800-342-2437.)

In February 1996, a judge in Austin, Texas, levied $915,000 in penalties against a water company. One witness against the company testified that the water from his faucet caught fire when he placed a candle near it.

The EPA makes water safety rules, and the states are responsible for enforcing them. However, they rarely take action against utilities in violation. When the states do not intervene, the EPA is supposed to step in. However, both federal and state agencies claim that they have insufficient funds to get tough against offenders. The General Accounting Office, the investigative branch of Congress, repeatedly finds problems. A 1990 investigation revealed that states take action against only one-fourth of the utilities that chronically violate EPA standards. They found that, of those water companies that violate standards, almost half of them do so for more than 4 years before any action is taken. Some of these violations pose serious health risks. In 1995 alone, close to 9,000 violations of contaminant levels in community drinking water were exposed.

It is important to drink *pure* water. Why do I stress pure water as opposed to just water? At a recent meeting of Health in Common, an organization of consumers and health-care providers, I had the opportunity to hear a presentation by Larry Colb from the California State Water Quality Control Board. When asked how many chemical substances California's state-of-the-art water treatment facilities test for, he told us "about seventy or so." Yet each year, as we learned from the U.S. Surgeon General as early as 1979, one thousand new man-made chemicals are released into the environment. Our modern water purification systems are testing for fewer than 10 percent of the possible pollutants that are produced annually. The seventy or so that are tested for also exclude the thousand or more chemicals that were introduced last year and the thousand or more produced and released the year before and the year before that.

The problem with water is even more insidious than synthetic chemicals in our environment winding up in our water supply because the chlorine that is used to disinfect drinking water is in itself harmful and dangerous when mixed with organic residues in the water we consume. Trihalomethanes (THMs) formed by the chemical bonding of chlorine with organic residues (such as dead leaves that drop into reservoirs) in water are known carcinogens:

- In rodent studies, THMs were carcinogenic in the liver, kidney, and/or intestines.[1]
- Landi and colleagues found a slightly elevated risk of cancer of the colon and bladder.[2]
- Human studies also indicate risk from the by-products of chlorination: "[V]arious toxicological and epidemiological studies point towards an association between THMs and low birth weight, spontaneous abortions, still births and birth defects."[3]
- Breast cancer has been implicated as a result of drinking chlorinated tap water.[4]

The EPA is aware of this problem and has set standards for levels of THMs that cannot be met in areas that have water supplies from reservoirs where dead leaves collect.

Because water treatment facilities are aware of the problem of trihalomethanes, some of them work to reduce THM levels by adding ammonia to the water after the chlorine has sat for a while. When ammonia is added, the chlorine preferentially bonds to the ammonia, thus reducing the formation of carcinogens. However, the ammonia-chlorine combination stays in the water longer than chlorine alone. This combination can cause problems for dialysis patients, rubber seals, gaskets, and some equipment—and it kills fish. Ammonia is also harder to take out of the water than chlorine is: Larger filters are required, the water must be in contact with the filter longer, and filters are fouled more quickly. With chlorine alone, the filter may last 3 years before it needs to be replaced; with ammonia present, the filter lasts only about 6 months. If the filter is not changed after 6 months, the THMs that were trapped by the carbon molecules may begin to release back into your water supply to trap new ammonia particles pouring through the filter.

For most people, these levels will not create an immediate health risk, but we simply don't know what the effect may be over time. For young, old, or sick populations, these small effects may add up to dysfunction and disease.

Toxic Plumbing

Next, we must consider the pipes that deliver water to our faucets and the material from which the faucets are made. There is concern about lead entering the water from solder and faucets. According to a February 1997 report from the EPA, 91 percent of the lead that contaminates domestic water is leached from the plumbing, rather than coming from the water source. Many people are familiar with the toxic effects that exposure to lead in house paints can have on childhood brain development, such as learning disabilities requiring remedial education, impaired visual-motor development, damage to the nervous and immune systems, and behavioral problems.

Some homes have copper water-supply pipes. Copper ions from the pipes can leach into the water supply. In a 1995 report, "The Need to Revise the National Drinking Water Regulations for Copper," K. S. Sidhu Prom recommended that the level of copper in our drinking water be reduced.[5] Infants and children up to 10 years old have an increased susceptibility to copper toxicity due to the presence of a normally high concentration of copper in their livers during early life and the lack of mechanisms to regulate it in their bodies. Adverse effects of copper toxicity are abdominal pain, nausea, vomiting, diarrhea, headaches, and dizziness.

Faced with the facts of poor water quality, point-of-use water filtration systems for your kitchen, shower, and bathtub faucets make sense. (For more information on water filters, see chapter 5 and appendix 1.)

TOXIC OVERLOAD

In September 1991, the EPA published a report entitled *Toxics in the Community: The 1989 Toxics Release Inventory (TRI) National Report,* which yielded some staggering figures. The largest toxic releases involved twenty-five chemicals, and totaled 5,705,670,380 pounds. Of this 5.7 billion pounds, 42.5 percent went into the air, 3.3 percent were released into surface water, 7.8 percent were on land, 20.7 percent flowed into underground water, 9.6 percent joined with public sewage, and 16 percent were off-site (brought to other places, such as surface impoundments). Among the twenty-five toxic substances were toluene, a known carcinogen commonly found in nail polish; sulfuric acid, a poison to lungs and mucous membranes; and freon, which destroys the ozone layer and causes increased exposure to excess ultraviolet rays, increasing the risk of skin cancer.

Although PCBs have been banned in the United States since 1976, nothing has been done to limit the use of PCBs already manufactured, so we continue to suffer the consequences of exposure. And dioxins continue to be released into our environment as a result of the production of pesticides and wood preservatives, bleaching paper to make it white, burning trash that contains plastics and paper, and burning fossil fuels (cooking and driving automobiles).

How to Avoid Dioxins

Don't despair. You can take immediate, effective steps to minimize or eliminate most risks of living in an industrialized world. Here are some alternatives to the dioxin-producing processes:

- Avoid the use of pesticides on your lawn, and talk to neighbors about doing the same.
- Ask your local hardware store to carry dioxin-free wood preservatives.
- Buy unbleached paper products for your kitchen and bathroom.
- If your trash is burned, separate out plastics and paper for recycling.
- Eat more raw fruits and vegetables if your digestion permits (if not, cook them as lightly as possible and/or consult a specialist to help you improve your digestion).
- Drive less, walk more, ride a bicycle, or carpool.

Toxic Agents of War

On March 15, 2000, the U.S. Air Force released The Statement on Results from the 1997 Physical Examination of the Ranch Hand Study (also known as the Ranch Hand Study). Dr. Joel Michalek, senior principal investigator for the Air Force Health Study on Agent Orange (Agent Orange, a dioxin, is an herbicide that was used in the Vietnam War that damaged the health of soldiers and civilians who were exposed) stated, "This report includes the strongest evidence to date that Agent Orange is associated with Adult Onset Diabetes based on 1997 exams." As dioxin levels went up, the severity of diabetes increased, and the time to onset decreased. There was a 47 percent increase in diabetes in people with the highest levels of dioxin. Other negative health effects reported were those to the heart and the nervous system. Increased blood pressure and heart attacks increased with dioxin levels, and soldiers suffered a loss of sensation in their feet.[6] In adult-onset diabetes, the body does not respond normally to insulin, a hormone that takes sugar out of your blood and puts it into your cells. As a result, levels of sugar in the blood rise, putting patients at risk for heart disease, kidney failure, and nerve damage. In a 1998 article that appeared in the *American Journal of Epidemiology*, Dr. Michalek reported that the Operation Ranch Hand Unit responsible for aerially spraying herbicides in Vietnam had "an increased number of deaths compared to vets in South East Asia not involved with spraying from cirrhosis, chronic liver disease and atherosclerotic heart disease."[7]

The soldiers' offspring were also put at risk. March 14, 1996, the Office of News and Public Information reported that "the father's exposure may put his children at a greater risk of being born with spina bifida, which is characterized by a deformity of the spinal cord and can cause neurologic problems." This possibility was also reported by Stephenson in the April 1996 issue of *JAMA*, the *Journal of the American Medical Association*.[8]

We are now seeing the negative health effects of agents used in Desert Storm. According to Dr. Jeffrey Bland, there were "an unexpected number of suicides in the returning vets who were still ill." Dr. Bland submitted a grant to the Veterans Department to help these unfortunate soldiers but it was never authorized. However, he informed me that "many of the men and women did get treatment through environmental medical doctors using HealthComm's mitochondrial resuscitation approach and detoxification with favorable results both symptomatically and biochemically. This concept still deserves a larger controlled study, I believe." The National Institute of Medicine is now studying the health effects associated with toxic exposure during the Persian Gulf War.

Hormone Disruption

In July 1991 a prestigious group of scientists—including experts in anthropology, ecology, toxicology, law, psychiatry, wildlife management, medicine, and related fields—met because they were concerned about the hormone-disrupting effects of substances like diethylstilbestrol (DES) in the environment. Their meeting produced what is called "The Wingspread Consensus Statement." On the subject of "Chemically-Induced Alterations in Sexual Development: The Wildlife/Human Connection," they stated with certainty that "[t]he effects seen in in utero DES-exposed humans parallel those found in contaminated wildlife and laboratory animals, suggesting that humans may be at risk to the same environmental hazards as wildlife."

Endocrine specialists have found little difference among the hormone functions of most species that inhabit the Earth. What happens to one species hormonally happens to all species. I interpret their statement to mean that we cannot ignore the disappearance of our Great Lakes mink populations or the problems observed in bird populations: eggs that don't hatch; deformities such as crossed bills, missing eyes, and clubbed feet; and abnormal nesting behavior. Nor can we ignore the fact that our St. Lawrence River beluga whale population is now a mere five hundred, down from five thousand at the turn of the century; that 80 percent of the sanderling bird population dropped in a 15-year period; and that half the population of bottlenose dolphins that migrate along the eastern seaboard were lost to sickness from pesticide-induced immune system suppression.

Some people explain the disappearance of wildlife from the planet with reasons other than xenobiotic poisoning, such as habitat destruction, overkill, and species competition. However, these reasons cannot account for the pathologies found during autopsy of dead fish, birds, and mammals. Autopsied beluga whales had malignant and benign tumors; breast tumors; abdominal masses; bladder cancer; emphysema; and ulcers of the mouth, esophagus, stomach, and intestines. Most had severe gum disease and missing teeth. Many had pneumonia or viral and bacterial infections. More than half of the females had breast infections that made it impossible to feed their young. Other beluga whales had endocrine disorders, including enlargement of the thyroid gland and cysts in the thyroid. Some had twisted spines and other skeletal disorders. Xenobiotic poisoning has been shown to be the cause of many of these disorders.

We live on this planet with those diseased and deformed fish, birds, and mammals. It is unlikely that we humans can escape exposure to the same environmental poisons that damage our wildlife, because we share the same Earth, air, and water.

Researchers disagree over whether environmental estrogens pose a threat to human health, but past episodes with compounds such as DES have led most to look carefully at these compounds. "Instead of assuming these chemicals to be safe until proven harmful, we should presume they have potential for harm," said Shanna Swan, Ph.D., chief of the Environmental Health Branch of the California Department of Health Services. Frederick S. Vomsaal, Ph.D., professor of biological sciences at the University of Missouri at Columbia, said that compounds such as methoxychlor and bisphenol A (found in plastics; see chapter 4) in amounts as small as parts per trillion—millions of times lower than current federal safety estimates—can affect a developing fetus.[9]

Recent newspaper articles report that breast cancer is reaching epidemic proportions. Considering women of all ages, one out of eight women will develop breast cancer in her lifetime. The most well-defined environmental risk factors are radiation exposure and alcohol ingestion. Diet is clearly related to the increased incidence in developed countries. Exposure to organochlorides, including DDT, is a recognized risk factor. In some studies, cigarette smoking is associated with greater risk among women who began smoking at an early age.[10] Several studies suggest an association with exposure to DDT.[11–13] Short-term exposure to TCDD, a dioxin, decreased uterine and breast cancer risk,[14] but long-term exposure elevated breast cancer mortality among women.[15,16] Moreover, environmental contaminants have other hormonal effects, including changes in gender, change in onset of puberty (earlier), and inhibition or promotion of tumor formation.[17]

Beginning in the San Francisco Bay area, the University of California–San Francisco, Alta Bates Medical Center in Berkeley, and California Pacific Medical Center in San Francisco are enrolling women with early and advanced breast cancer into studies with Chinese and Tibetan herbs. They will be analyzing whether these promising herbal preparations ease the effects of chemotherapy, kill cancer cells, or shrink tumors.

Unlike our unfortunate wildlife, we have a surer way to aid recovery: detoxification.

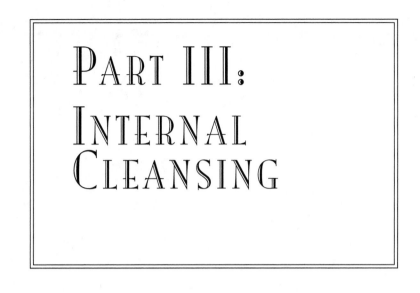

PART III:
INTERNAL
CLEANSING

DIETARY FIBER FOR GOOD HEALTH

My grandmother used to tell me to eat my roughage (also called crude fiber—the cellulose or cell wall of plants). Scientists have found other equally active components of fiber, including cellulose, hemicellulose, pectin, lignan, gums, and mucilages. Dietary fiber has been defined as the substances in food that are not digested and absorbed in the small intestines.

The FDA has set a Recommended Daily Allowance (RDA) for dietary fiber of 25 grams per day for a 2,000-calorie diet. If you take in less or more than 2,000 calories a day, as many Americans do, they recommend adjusting the amount of fiber accordingly. The standard Western diet contains only 10 to 20 grams of fiber per day, while research points to the necessity of at least 40 to 60 grams per day for good health. Bad habits start young. According to Dr. Christine Williams from the Columbia University Children's Hospital, New York, 89 percent of adolescents in the United States are not getting the recommended amount of dietary fiber. (The most current scientific recommendation for child fiber intake is to take the child's age and add 5 grams of fiber to that number. For example, a 10 year old would need 15 grams of fiber per day.)[1] The FDA came only halfway with its recommendation for optimal fiber intake, but it is a definite improvement over no recommendation at all. Low fiber intake is one of the reasons there is such an urgent need for internal cleansing in Western countries.

Fiber comes in many forms. For most people, the best way to get adequate fiber is to eat lots of fruit and vegetables. Sadly, most Americans get most of their fiber from white bread. Knowing this, it is not surprising to learn that Americans are sorely deficient in this important dietary component. In their book *The Omega-3 Phenomenon*, nutritionist Clara Felix and Donald Rudin, M.D., note that the fiber content of white bread is less than one gram per slice. The American Dietetic Association, The National Institutes of Health, and the American Cancer Society recommend five to nine servings of fruits and vegetables per day. The National Cancer Institute defines a serving as a medium piece of fruit, ½ cup fruit or vegetable, ¾ cup (6 ounces) juice, 1 cup leafy greens, or ¼ cup dried fruit. To simplify you might use the Health Coach version: One serving equals one cup of raw, or one-half cup of cooked, fruit or vegetables. Those who eat up to ten servings per day are even more healthy than those who eat only five servings per day. In this case more is better.

In summarizing their review of the scientific literature on dietary fiber, Martin A. Eastwood and R. Passmore, fiber researchers who followed up on Dr. Denis Burkitt's work, concluded in the *Lancet:* "It can be stated with confidence that people who increase their fiber intake up to 50 grams per day [which is] double the amount usually present in

British [and other Western] diets run no risk of any serious adverse effects on their health." Some reports have stated that very high-fiber diets, especially those with high wheat bran content, may tend to bind some minerals and thus reduce their absorption in the body.

FIBER SUPPLEMENTS

If you are concerned about mineral absorption, choose fiber supplements other than wheat bran. I use three fiber supplements in my office: Colon Care Formula (CCF) by Yerba Prima, Meta Fiber (MF) by Metagenics, and Nutri Flax (NF) by Omega Nutrition. Colon Care Formula and Meta Fiber are combinations of soluble and insoluble fibers for optimal effect. Meta Fiber has no psyllium husks in it for persons who have a sensitivity to this form of fiber. It does, however, have a high concentration of barley fiber, which can be problematic for some sensitive individuals. Nutri Flax is powdered flaxseed that has been specially prepared to ensure freshness and effectiveness. If there is a concern regarding cancer risk, this would be my fiber of choice since flax fiber promotes the production of mammalian lignan, which has a potent anticancer effect. It is very helpful to have three high-quality therapeutic options for people who need a fiber supplement.

Fiber Improves Bowel Function

With an increase in daily fiber intake, you will typically be immediately aware of an improvement in bowel function. Dietary fiber—in particular the hemicellulose portion—absorbs water in the intestines to provide bulk and soften the stools. This makes for less straining with bowel movements. The hemicellulose type of fiber is essential because of its ability to absorb released toxins and aid in elimination from the body.

Fiber Decreases Transit Time

Increased daily fiber intake will decrease the time it takes for the food you eat to pass through your 20 to 30 feet of intestinal tubing and be eliminated in a bowel movement. It takes approximately 10 hours for food to pass into the colon, but the amount of time it sits in the colon can vary dramatically. While the normal range of total transit time for people on a high-fiber diet is 10 to 50 hours, people on a Western diet have an average transit time of 65 to 100 hours. For most of those hours, the partially digested food (now your body's waste material) sits in the colon being worked on by disease-producing yeasts and bacteria. Normal transit time is a health blessing because environmental and dietary toxins have less time to come in contact with the colon lining and therefore less chance to be reabsorbed into your bloodstream (see Figure 2.1).

Fiber Normalizes the Bowel

Paradoxically, fiber is also helpful for people who have an irritable bowel with loose, frequent, and perhaps urgent bowel movements. It helps both with constipation or sluggish bowel movements and diarrhea or loose bowel movements.

Fiber Lowers Cholesterol Levels

Studies have shown that some fibers, such as psyllium husks, pectin, oat and rice bran, and guar gum, have a cholesterol-lowering effect on the blood. They lower the level of harmful LDL cholesterol in the body, while raising the valuable and protective HDL cholesterol level. One man I know found that after daily use of psyllium husks for 4 months (2 teaspoons per day), his cholesterol count dropped from 260 to under 200, the lowest it had ever been. This change in his cholesterol from the simple addition of dietary fiber took his heart attack risk back down into the normal range.

Fiber Protects Against Chronic Degenerative Disease

Over the years, daily fiber intake will protect against the risk of a number of chronic diseases. Its antitoxic properties, its ability to nourish the growth of beneficial intestinal bacteria such as lactobacillus, its sweeping action in the colon, and its swelling action, which results in softer and bulkier stools, all contribute to long-term health. Research findings worldwide led the director of the Division of Cancer Prevention and Control at the National Cancer Institute to issue a statement in August of 1984 recommending that Americans eat a diet high in fiber to reduce the risk of colon and rectal cancer. In 1992, colon and rectal cancer were the third leading cause of death. In 2000, these types of cancer were the second leading cause of death as published in an article about colon cancer in the March 13, 2000, issue of *Time* magazine. It is becoming ever more important to take good care of our intestinal tracts. Heart disease may also be prevented by eating five to nine servings of fruits and vegetables per day both because of their antioxidant content as well as their high-fiber content according to a June 2000 article by J. H. Weisberger in the *American Journal of Clinical*

Nutrition. The many benefits of dietary fiber are summarized in Figure 3.2.

Fiber Normalizes Blood Sugar

Fiber slows the release of sugar into your bloodstream, which prevents an exhausting demand for the release of insulin. If you have normal pancreatic function, your body produces insulin in response to the sugar load in your bloodstream from food you have eaten. Insulin brings your blood levels back into a normal range. Diabetics who cannot produce insulin from their pancreas must use medication in tablet form or by injection to normalize their blood sugar. As a benefit of adequate fiber intake, insulin-dependent diabetics may be able to reduce their required dose of insulin. If you do have diabetes, decrease your insulin intake only under the supervision of your medical doctor to assure your safety. Hypoglycemic individuals can maintain a more stable blood sugar level and prevent peaks and valleys in their daily energy by including more fiber in their diet.

Fiber and Breast Cancer

Scientific studies show that a high-fiber diet can reduce breast cancer risk. Rose and her colleagues speculated that this may be due, at least in part, to the reduction in circulating estrogens. Elevating fiber levels to 20 to 32 grams per day resulted in a significant reduction in estrogens after 2 months.[2]

There are two broad types of fiber, soluble and insoluble. Soluble fibers are present in fruits and vegetables and certain grains such as oats. Soluble fiber is food for intestinal bacteria. The metabolized by-products of soluble fiber detoxify colon carcinogens thus reducing cancer-causing agents in your large intestines. Insoluble fiber increases stool size in several ways including water retention. This larger bulk dilutes carcinogens resulting in lower risk of colon cancer and to a lesser extent breast cancer in animals and humans.[3]

In earlier research, Rose discovered that, "Based on present evidence, a dietary approach to breast cancer prevention should include weight control, when indicated, a reduction in dietary fat to approximately 20 percent of total fats, and an increase in fiber consumption to 25–30 grams per day."[4]

A shortened menstrual cycle (less than 24 days) is known to correlate with an increased risk of breast cancer. A 1994 study showed that dietary fiber lengthened the menstrual cycle by almost 1 day.[5]

African-American women have a diminished 5-year survival rate from breast cancer compared to Caucasian women, 69 versus 84 percent respectively. Because estrogen levels are known to be a risk factor for breast cancer and a low fat, high fiber diet is known to reduce estrogen levels, Woods and team analyzed estrogen levels in African-American women after a 3-week trial on their usual diet of high fat (40 percent) and low fiber (12 grams per day). After testing, their estrogen levels were elevated compared to Caucasian women. After a diet consisting of a low level of fat (only 20 percent) and high fiber (40 grams per day) for two menstrual cycles, they were retested. The investigators found that dietary modification can result in the lowering of serum estrogens.[6]

A HISTORY OF
BREAKFAST FIBER IN AMERICA

The history of modern interest in good nutrition as it relates to health is intertwined with fiber cereals and eating a good breakfast. This is hard to imagine when you step into the cereal aisle of your local supermarket. Row after row of bright, colorful, sugar-laden cereals nearly jump off the shelves and into your cart. When children are along on a shopping trip, the sugar cereals they have seen advertised on their cartoon shows usually succeed in making it into the cart. Of course, adults are not immune to this siren call. Yet more adults are picking up high-fiber cereals such as Kellogg's All Bran, Post Raisin Bran, Quaker Oat Bran, and various rice bran cereals. This brings us back to our nineteenth-century roots.

Breakfast was not always considered a distinct meal. The first concepts of breakfast date back to the 1400s. Then it was usually a high-fat, high-calorie meal geared toward heavy agricultural or manual labor. Agricultural workers may have been able to use up all of those calories throughout the day, but can you?

The transition took place over time in the 1800s and early 1900s. Graham crackers are named after health pioneer Sylvester Graham, who in the mid-1800s stressed the importance of whole-meal bread with the fiber intact. Seventh Day Adventists followed up on Graham's teachings. One very influential advocate, Sister Ellen White, began the Battle Creek Sanitarium in Battle Creek, Michigan, in the late 1800s. She taught the value of whole grains and vegetarian diet for good health. One of the early whole grain cereals served at the sanitarium was called Granose Flakes.

Two of the employees at the Battle Creek Sanitarium were W. K. Kellogg and John Harvey Kellogg. In the world of cereals, there is no name more famous than Kellogg. The Kellogg company began in 1906 with Kellogg's Corn Flakes. To this day, Kellogg's Corn Flakes remains the top-selling cereal in the world. Their best-known high-fiber cereal, All Bran, began in 1916 as Krumbled Bran and was changed to its current name in 1923. You and I both know why people eat All Bran. Until 1941, the label was quite explicit: It said right on the box, "Relieves Constipation."

Kellogg's All Bran is known for one more breakthrough, though, in the 1980s. With the cooperation of the National Cancer Institute, Kellogg's began an educational campaign on the back of All Bran boxes describing the link between high-fiber diets and reduced risk of cancer. Sales of All Bran doubled, while the FDA objected to these claims. This pioneering move by Kellogg's in their eighth decade helped pave the way for the Nutrition Labeling and Education Act of 1990 and the Dietary Supplement Health and Education Act of 1994. Despite FDA objections and because there was such a positive response from both consumers and health professionals to the information linking fiber and a decreased risk of colon cancer, legislators were pressured to ensure more health education information on product labels.

Since then, Kellogg's has experimented with psyllium cereal to lower cholesterol levels. They have not been commercially successful, but Quaker has been successful with its oatmeal and oat bran products. Quaker began working with Dr. James Anderson at the University of Kentucky over two decades ago, studying the cholesterol-lowering properties of oatmeal. Over the years, they determined that the soluble portion of oat bran, also called beta glucan, is responsible for lowering cholesterol levels. Recently, Quaker became the first company to receive approval from the FDA for its health claim because the oat-soluble fiber research is so solid. We look at oat bran in more detail in chapter 9.

CHAPTER 8

THE BASICS OF INTERNAL CLEANSING

Internal cleansing works in the same way that natural hygiene works on the outside of your body. Your body uses the colon, skin, lungs, and other organs to eliminate toxins as quickly as possible. If these systems are sluggish or overburdened, the toxins back up into your body and cause headaches, loss of energy, fatigue, aches and pains, and a host of other maladies. Years of improper elimination can lead to the most severe health problems. Internal cleansing is a preventive means to assist your body in keeping its channels of elimination open and clean so that they can perform their vital functions.

The practice of cleansing has existed for thousands of years and has played a central role in the lives of millions of people throughout the world. The Greeks, Romans, Japanese, Turks, Finns, and Russians have all had a form of sauna or bathhouse that played a central role in both their medical practices and social lives. These baths incorporated both sweating and skin brushing as methods to rid the body of stored toxins. The American Indians used their sweat lodges in much the same way. The understanding behind these practices was that cleansing the body of built-up toxins would promote health and prevent degenerative disease. Semiannual trips to the local spa are still a common practice among Europeans.

Dr. Hulda Regehr Clark, author of *The Cure for All Diseases*, points out that all over the world people perform annual cleansing rituals, generally in the spring. In colonial America, people did a sulfur and molasses "cure." In modern America, however, we are lulled into a false sense of security by believing that we are protected from nasty microbes.

Do you need internal cleansing? Look again at the "Autointoxication Checklist" in the Introduction, as well as Figure 8.1, the Metabolic Screening Questionnaire, and Figure 8.2, the Dysbiosis Questionnaire and Score Sheet. These tools will help you evaluate your need for some type of internal cleansing program.

In working with patients and training with colleagues, researchers, and scientists over the years, I have developed and promoted several cleansing programs for increasing health and vitality. As I do with my patients and clients, I offer here a number of options to meet your health, time, and budgetary needs. Cleansing products are available in health food stores all over the world; you can purchase and most likely self-administer them safely. Remember, if you are pregnant or have serious health problems, consult first with a health-care practitioner before engaging in any cleansing program. It is generally best to work with a trained professional who can support your specific needs, put you in touch with the best products, perform diagnostic work,

Figure 8.1 Metabolic Screening Questionnaire

Patient Name _____ Date _____ Week _____

Rate each of the following symptoms
based upon your typical health profile for:
☐ Past 30 days   ☐ Past 48 hours

Point Scale: 0 = *Never or almost never* have the symptom
1 = *Occasionally* have it, effect is *not severe*
2 = *Occasionally* have it, effect is *severe*
3 = *Frequently* have it, effect is *not severe*
4 = *Frequently* have it, effect is *severe*

HEAD _____ Headaches
_____ Faintness
_____ Dizziness
_____ Insomnia   **Total** _____

EYES _____ Watery or itchy eyes
_____ Swollen, reddened, or sticky eyelids
_____ Bags or dark circles under eyes
_____ Blurred or tunnel vision (does not
include near- or far-sightedness)   **Total** _____

EARS _____ Itchy ears
_____ Earaches, ear infections
_____ Drainage from ear
_____ Ringing in ears, hearing loss   **Total** _____

NOSE _____ Stuffy nose
_____ Sinus problems
_____ Hay fever
_____ Sneezing attacks
_____ Excessive mucus formation   **Total** _____

MOUTH/ _____ Chronic coughing
THROAT _____ Gagging, frequent need to clear
throat
_____ Sore throat, hoarseness, loss of
voice
_____ Swollen or discolored tongue,
gums, lips
_____ Canker sores   **Total** _____

SKIN _____ Acne
_____ Hives, rash, dry skin
_____ Hair loss
_____ Flushing, hot flashes
_____ Excessive sweating   **Total** _____

Continues

Figure 8.1   (continued)

HEART	_____ Irregular or skipped heartbeat	
	_____ Rapid or pounding heartbeat	
	_____ Chest pain	**Total** _____
LUNGS	_____ Chest congestion	
	_____ Asthma, bronchitis	
	_____ Shortness of breath	
	_____ Difficulty breathing	**Total** _____
DIGESTIVE TRACT	_____ Nausea, vomiting	
	_____ Diarrhea	
	_____ Constipation	
	_____ Bloated feeling	
	_____ Belching, passing gas	
	_____ Heartburn	
	_____ Intestinal/stomach pain	**Total** _____
JOINTS/ MUSCLE	_____ Pain or aches in joints	
	_____ Arthritis	
	_____ Stiffness or limitation of movement	
	_____ Pain or aches in muscles	
	_____ Feeling of weakness or tiredness	**Total** _____
WEIGHT	_____ Binge eating/drinking	
	_____ Craving certain foods	
	_____ Excessive weight	
	_____ Compulsive eating	
	_____ Water retention	
	_____ Underweight	**Total** _____
ENERGY/ ACTIVITY	_____ Fatigue, sluggishness	
	_____ Apathy, lethargy	
	_____ Hyperactivity	
	_____ Restlessness	**Total** _____
MIND	_____ Poor memory	
	_____ Confusion, poor comprehension	
	_____ Poor concentration	
	_____ Poor physical coordination	
	_____ Difficulty in making decisions	
	_____ Stuttering or stammering	
	_____ Slurred speech	
	_____ Learning disabilities	**Total** _____

EMOTIONS	_____ Mood swings	
	_____ Anxiety, fear, nervousness	
	_____ Anger, irritability, aggressiveness	
	_____ Depression	**Total** _____
OTHER	_____ Frequent illness	
	_____ Frequent or urgent urination	
	_____ Genital itch or discharge	**Total** _____
GRAND TOTAL		**GRAND TOTAL** _____

If you score 10 points or higher for any individual section or have a grand total of 50 points or more, you should seek the help of a health-care practitioner.

Reprinted by permission of HealthComm International, Inc.

keep you on track, monitor your progress, and help you through rough spots.

FASTING

Fasting has been used by many cultures as a way of cleansing the body's internal systems. However, fasting can damage the digestive system by starving the microvilli, because their preferred food comes from the inside of your gut. Furthermore, during an extended fast you may lose lean body mass, which would cause wasting of your vital organs. Researchers, using rats to discover what effect fasting has on a body, found that the liver has a decreased ability to detoxify pesticides and drugs as early as 36 hours into the fast.

A short fast using pure water and freshly made fruit and/or vegetable juice may allow your body to receive nutrition and avoid starving your digestive lining while giving your system a rest from the work of breaking down large amounts of food into absorbable nutrients. A juice fast, however, may prove harmful to

Figure 8.2   Dysbiosis Questionnaire and Score Sheet

This questionnaire is designed for adults and the scoring system isn't as appropriate for children. It lists factors in your medical history that are known to contribute to the disruption of normal healthy gastrointestinal bacteria, directly or indirectly promoting the overgrowth of yeasts, fungi, and other pathogens (Section A) and symptoms commonly found in individuals with dysbiosis related illness (Sections B and C).

For each "Yes" answer in Section A, circle the Point Score in that section. Total your score and record it in the box at the end of the section. Then move on to Sections B and C and score as directed.

Filling out and scoring this questionnaire should help you and your physician evaluate the possible role of dysbiosis in contributing to your health problems. Yet it will not provide an automatic "Yes" or "No" answer.

NOTE: **Dysbiosis refers to the condition where the normal healthy population of beneficial bacteria in the intestines has been disrupted, leaving it open to the overgrowth of yeast, fungi, parasites, and potentially harmful strains of bacteria. This intestinal imbalance in turn adversely affects other important organ systems via toxic stress and interfering with nutrient absorption and utilization.**

Section A: History	Point Score
1. Have you taken tetracyclines (Sumycin, Panmycin, Vibramycin, Minocin, etc.) or other antibiotics for skin, acne, or anything else for 1 month (or longer)?	25
2. Have you, *at any time in your life,* taken other "broad spectrum" antibiotics for respiratory, urinary, or other infections in shorter courses 4 or more times in a 1 year period?	20
3. Have you taken a broad spectrum antibiotic drug — even in a single course?	6
4. Have you, at any time in your life, been bothered by recurrent or persistent prostatitis, vaginitis, or other problems affecting your reproductive organs?	25

5. Have you taken birth control pills . . .
   - For more than 5 years? ... 25
   - For more than 2 years? ... 15
   - For 6 months to 2 years? ... 8

6. Have you been pregnant . . .
   - 2 or more times? ... 5
   - 1 time? ... 3

7. Have you taken prednisone, Decadron, or other cortisone type drugs . . .
   - For more than 6 months? ... 25
   - For more than 2 weeks? ... 15
   - For 2 weeks or less? ... 6

8. Does exposure to perfumes, insecticides, fabric shop odors, and other chemicals provoke . . .
   - Moderate to severe symptoms? ... 20
   - Mild symptoms? ... 5
   - List symptoms:

9. Are your symptoms worse on damp, muggy days or in moldy places? ... 20
   - List symptoms:

10. Have you had athlete's foot, ring worm, "jock itch," or other chronic fungus infections of the skin or nails? ... Y/N
    Have such infections been
    - Severe or persistant? ... 20
    - Mild to moderate? ... 10

11. Do you crave sugar? ... 10

12. Do you crave breads? ... 10

13. Do you crave alcoholic beverages? ... 10

14. Does tobacco smoke really bother you? ... 10

15. Have you ever had parasitic infection, dysentery, or an unexplained episode of prolonged diarrhea and/or intestinal distress? ... 15

Continues

Figure 8.2   (continued)

16. Have you ever consumed chlorinated (or chemically treated) drinking water for 3 or more months?	15
17. Do you consume commercially raised flesh foods (antibiotic fed) on a regular basis?	15
18. Do you eat processed foods regularly?	20
19. Do you drink alcohol or consume coffee daily?	20
20. Do you have or have you ever had an ulcer, colitis, Crohn's disease, or diverticulitis?	35
21. Were you breast fed? If no.	35
If yes, but for less than 3 months.	20

Total Score, Section A   _____

Section B: Major Symptoms   Point Score

For each of your symptoms, enter the appropriate figure in the Point Score column:

    If a symptom is occasional or mild, score 3 points

    If a symptom is frequent and/or moderately severe, score 6 points

    If a symptom is severe and/or disabling, score 9 points

Add total score and record it in the box at the end of this section.

  1. Fatigue or lethargy   _____

  2. Feeling of being "drained"   _____

  3. Poor memory   _____

  4. Feeling "spacey" or "unreal"   _____

  5. Depression   _____

  6. Numbness, burning, or tingling   _____

  7. Muscle aches   _____

  8. Muscle weakness or paralysis   _____

  9. Pain and/or swelling in joints   _____

10. Abdominal pain   _____

11. Constipation   _____

12. Diarrhea   _____

13. Bloating   _____

14. Troublesome vaginal discharge   _____

15. Persistent vaginal burning or itching   _____

16. Prostatitis _____

17. Impotence _____

18. Loss of sexual desire _____

19. Endometriosis _____

20. Cramps and/or other menstrual irregularities _____

21. Premenstrual tension _____

22. Spots in front of eyes _____

23. Erratic vision _____

24. Eczema, dermatitis, psoriasis _____

Total Score, Section B _____

Section C: Other Symptoms   Point Score

For each of your symptoms, enter the appropriate figure in the Point Score column:

    If a symptom is occasional or mild score 3 points.

    If a symptom is frequent and/or moderately severe score 6 points.

    If a symptom is severe and/or disabling score 9 points.

Add total score and record it in the box at the end of this section.

1. Drowsiness _____

2. Irritability or jitteriness _____

3. Incoordination _____

4. Inability to concentrate _____

5. Frequent mood swings _____

6. Headache _____

7. Dizziness/loss of balance _____

8. Pressure above ears . . . feeling of head swelling and tingling _____

9. Itching _____

10. Other rashes _____

11. Heartburn _____

12. Indigestion _____

13. Belching and intestinal gas _____

14. Mucus in stools _____

Continues

Figure 8.2   (continued)

15. Hemorrhoids	_____
16. Dry mouth	_____
17. Rash or blisters in mouth	_____
18. Bad breath	_____
19. Nasal congestion or discharge	_____
20. Joint swelling or arthritis	_____
21. Postnasal drip	_____
22. Nasal itching	_____
23. Sore or dry throat	_____
24. Cough	_____
25. Pain or tightness in the chest	_____
26. Wheezing or shortness of breath	_____
27. Urgency or urinary frequency	_____
28. Burning on urination	_____
29. Failing vision	_____
30. Burning or tearing of eyes	_____
31. Recurrent infection or fluid in ears	_____
32. Ear pain or hearing loss	_____
Total Score, Section C	_____
Total Score, Section A	_____
Total Score, Section B	_____

Grand Total Score	_____

The Grand Total Score will help you and your physician decide if your health problems are dysbiosis related. Scores in women will run higher as 7 items in the questionnaire apply exclusively to women, while only 2 apply exclusively to men.

Dysbiosis related health problems are almost certainly present in women with scores over 180, and in men with scores over 140.

Dysbiosis related health problems are probably present in women with scores over 120 and in men with scores over 80.

With scores of less than 60 in women and 40 in men, dysbiosis is unlikely to be contributing to your health challenges.

those who are carbohydrate-intolerant. To find out if you are carbohydrate-intolerant, fill out the questionnaire "Determining Your Sensitivity to Insulinogenic Foods and Eating Habits." Answer yes or no to each question. The higher your score, the more careful you should be regarding your protein-to-carbohydrate ratio at each meal.

Determining Your Sensitivity to Insulinogenic Foods and Eating Habits

(5) _____ I have a tendency toward high blood pressure.

(5) _____ I gain weight easily, especially around my waist, and I have difficulty losing it.

(5) _____ I often experience mental confusion.

(5) _____ I often experience fatigue and generalized weakness.

(10) _____ I have diabetic tendencies.

(4) _____ I get tired and/or hungry in the mid-afternoon.

(5) _____ About an hour or two after eating a full meal that includes dessert, I want more of the dessert.

(3) _____ It is harder for me to control my eating for the rest of the day if I have a breakfast containing carbohydrates than it would be if I had only coffee or nothing at all.

(4) _____ When I want to lose weight, I find it easier not to eat for most of the day than to try to eat several small diet meals.

(3) _____ Once I start eating sweets, starches, or snack foods, I often have a difficult time stopping.

(3) _____ I would rather have an ordinary meal that included dessert than a gourmet meal that did not include dessert.

Continues

(5) _____ After finishing a full meal, I sometimes feel as if I could go back and eat the whole meal again.

(3) _____ A meal of only meat and vegetables leaves me feeling unsatisfied.

(3) _____ If I'm feeling down, a snack of cake or cookies makes me feel better.

(3) _____ If potatoes, bread, pasta, or dessert are on the table, I will often skip eating vegetables or salad.

(4) _____ I get a sleepy, almost "drugged" feeling after eating a large meal containing bread, pasta, or potatoes and dessert, whereas I feel more energetic after a meal of only meat or fish and salad.

(3) _____ Sometimes I have a hard time going to sleep without a bedtime snack.

(3) _____ Sometimes I wake in the middle of the night and can't go back to sleep unless I eat something.

(5) _____ I get irritable if I miss a meal or if mealtime is delayed.

(2) _____ At a restaurant, I almost always eat too much bread, even before the meal is served.

Total _____ (Add up the scores from the left of every question to which you answered "yes.")

SCORE: 1–20, eat a lowfat/high complex carbohydrate diet;
      25 or more, eat a modified low carbohydrate diet

There are studies indicating a need for the amino acid support provided by protein for adequate detoxification of xenobiotics. You may not get the protein you need from a water/juice fast. The Carbohydrate Classifications of Fruits and Vegetables charts list the carbohydrate content of fruits and vegetables. Many people who are carbohydrate-intolerant will find relief from their symptoms just by minimizing grains in their diet without having to consider the carbohydrate content of fruits and vegetables. If that is a factor, which only you can tell through experimentation, it would be wise to choose fruits and vegetables according to their carbohydrate content.

Carbohydrate Classifications of Vegetables (According to Carbohydrate Content)

3%	6%	15%	20%	25%
Asparagus	Beans, String	Artichokes	Beans, Dried	Potato,
Bean Sprouts	Beets	Carrots	Beans, Lima	Sweet
Beet Greens	Brussels	Oyster Plant	Corn	Yams
Broccoli	Sprouts	Parsnips	Potato, White	
Cabbage	Chives	Peas, Green		
Cauliflower	Collard	Squash		
Celery	Greens			
Chard, Swiss	Dandelion			
Cucumber	Greens			
Endive	Eggplant			
Lettuce	Kale			
Mustard	Kohlrabi			
Greens	Leeks			
Radishes	Onions			
Spinach	Parsley			
Watercress	Peppers, Red			
	Pimento			
	Pumpkin			
	Rutabagas			
	Turnip			

Here are some guidelines for a lower carbohydrate program:

- Eat all of the 3% and 6% vegetable selections that you wish, and the 15% to 25% vegetables in limited quantities. Include only one type of the 15% to 25% vegetables at each meal; they are nutritious and should generally be part of your diet unless your Health Coach has told you otherwise.

- Eat fruit separately from other foods, and preferably in the morning. Choose limited quantities of the 3% or 6% fruit daily, eating a small amount (one cup) at any one time; watch for intolerance to citrus fruit and melons. The 15% to 20% fruits may be selected, but only in small portions at any given time (such as ½ banana or 1 small apple or 3 prunes).
- Eat a large variety of foods, including many different types, but rotate them as much as possible. Avoid eating the same foods day after day.

Carbohydrate Classifications of Fruits (According to Carbohydrate Content)

3 %	6 %	15 %	20 %	25 %
Cantaloupe	Apricots	Apples	Bananas	
Melons	(fresh only)	Blueberries	Figs	
Rhubarb	Blackberries	Cherries	Prunes	
Strawberries	Cranberries	Grapes	or any	
Tomatoes	Grapefruit	Kumquats	dried	
Watermelon	Guava	Loganberries	fruits	
	Kiwis	Mangoes		
	Lemons	Mulberries		
	Limes	Pears		
	Oranges	Pineapple (fresh)		
	Papayas	Pomegranates		
	Peaches			
	Plums			
	Raspberries			
	Tangerines			

Reprinted by permission Health Coach Systems International, Inc., and New Health Perspectives.

If you lose fat during a fast, you will significantly reduce the toxic load that has accumulated in your body over the years, because most toxins are stored in the fatty tissue in your body.

But as you shed fat, those toxins are released into your system. What happens if you don't have adequate antioxidants to trap those nasty chemicals that come careening into your healthy cells for a second time? You get sick, you hurt, you don't have any energy, and so on. Refer to appendix 4 to test your level of oxidative stress and appendix 1 for nutrients that quench these damaging particles.

It's difficult to tell from which of your body tissues you are losing weight by looking in the mirror, trying on tight clothes, or standing on a scale. The weight you lose may be healthy lean tissue if your protein intake is not great enough. During a fast or cleansing program, it is advisable to have your body composition monitored with a bio-impedance system to ensure that you are not losing healthy tissue and that you are instead losing fat and excess water. (Many Health Coaches have this technology in their offices.)

A FOOD ONLY NINE-WEEK CLEANSING PROGRAM

A simple nine-week cleansing program recommended by Health Coach and naturopath Charley Cropley is to eat a minimum of two servings of fruits, three of vegetables, and one of a whole grain each day for three weeks. These foods form the backbone of your food choices. Add other foods such as clean protein—organic meat; cage free, organic eggs and poultry; deep, cold water fish; and organic soy products—as needed and desired. During the next three weeks, continue with the fruits, vegetables, and grain and choose, in addition, 3 consecutive days during the three-week period in which you eat only fruits and vegetables. During the last three weeks, continue with the fruit, vegetables, and grain, and choose 3 consecutive days during which you have only liquids. The liquid diet can consist of fresh fruit and/or vegetable juice and vegetable soup or broth.

Fruits, in general, tend to accelerate cleansing. If your cleansing is going too fast and you are experiencing uncomfortable symptoms, use more vegetables and less fruit. I have included a recipe for Alkaline Broth in chapter 13 that is nourishing during this three-day cleanse. Some of you may not do well with this program because of the low protein content, but it is simple, inexpensive, and easy to try. During the first 3 to 5 days of a cleanse, some people experience symptoms of a cold or flu. If you have these symptoms and they are severe or persist for longer than 5 days, then consult with your health-care practitioner.

Dr. Jeffrey Bland has developed a number of powdered therapeutic food products to support healing of the intestinal tract and detoxification of the liver; they can also help you lose fat and protect against losing protein from your muscles and organs. (For more information on Dr. Bland's detoxification program, see chapter 10.) These therapeutic foods are available in the offices of licensed health-care professionals.

Many Health Coaches have been specially trained to take you through cleansing programs using a modified elimination diet and these healing foods. Any fasting or cleansing program should be monitored carefully because a drastic cleansing can release toxins too quickly and cause severe reactions.

HERBS

Herbs were the first medicines, and according to the April 2000 issue of *National Geographic,* "Still, almost two-thirds of the Earth's 6.1 billion people rely on the healing power of plants." Also approximately half of our modern drugs were originally derived from herbs. In my practice, I find that herbs have profound healing abilities without causing many of the insidious side effects of modern synthesized drugs. I utilize chiropractic and herbal healing because both work with the whole person, seeking not only to address specific health complaints but also to accelerate my patients' and clients' progress toward optimal health.

Americans use of nonprescription botanical formulas is rising dramatically. According to the *National Geographic* article mentioned previously, "In 1990, 2.5 percent of Americans purchased herbal remedies; in 1997, 12.1 percent spent roughly five billion dollars on them." They quote Dr. Arnold Relman, editor in chief of the *New England Journal of Medicine* as saying, "Many plant derived materials have been proved to have important biological effects."[1]

In looking for a good herbal cleansing product, it is most important that the amounts and kinds of herbs interact properly. A formula should be designed so that the herbs work together to promote cleansing and avoid unpleasant reactions. In chapter 9, I will discuss a program that does just that.

CHAPTER 9

An Herb and Fiber Cleansing Program

The benefit of herb and fiber programs is that you cleanse your body without dramatically changing your current diet. This is the preferred method for many people who wish to decrease their toxic burden without making big lifestyle changes. My favorite program in this regard is the Yerba Prima Internal Cleansing Program; it is based on ancient traditions of herbal cleansing, yet it suits today's busy lifestyles. I recommend that my patients follow this cleansing program twice a year and maintain their colon during the rest of the year with a good diet and high-quality fiber supplements between cleansings. The program incorporates herbal formulas, in capsule form, called Herbal Guard, Men's Rebuild or Women's Renew, and a fiber cleansing formula called Prima Cleanse.

THE YERBA PRIMA
INTERNAL CLEANSING PROGRAM

The three requirements for optimum, vibrant health are a clean system, good digestion, and absorption of nutrients. The first step is a clean system. The Internal Cleansing Program supports the elimination organs to more completely remove toxins and waste from the body. It also reduces the reabsorption of toxins from the colon into the bloodstream, protecting against autointoxication. The Internal Cleansing Program promotes regularity in bowel movements and supports healthy liver function—both vital aspects of a healthy digestive system free of toxic buildup. It also helps remove parasites that can live in the body and cause numerous health problems.

REBUILDING DIGESTIVE FUNCTION

The second and third steps toward optimum health are rebuilding the digestive function and improving absorption of nutrients. Herbs in Herbal Guard, Men's Rebuild, and Women's Renew help promote healthy liver, kidney, small intestine, and colon function. They work with Prima Cleanse to promote energy production and rebuilding on a cellular level. They are designed to promote better nutrient absorption so that you get the most from the foods and supplements you eat. They also support the growth of friendly bacteria and help keep harmful bacteria and yeast populations in balance in your intestines.

The ingredients in the program help the following eliminative and digestive organs and systems: stomach, small intestines, colon, liver, gallbladder, kidneys and urinary system, lymphatic system, respiratory system, skin, and circulatory system. They have the following effects: cleansing, building healthy tissue, antioxidant protection, adaptogenic action (helping you to adapt to physical and mental stresses), improving digestion, improving assimilation, carminative action (expelling gas to relieve colic and griping—sharp pains in the bowels), removing parasites, removing toxins, probiotic action (promoting the growth of healthy intestinal factors), and renewing energy.

Women's Renew, Men's Rebuild, and Herbal Guard

To meet the different needs of men and women, Yerba Prima modified Kalenite, the original formula, to make it more gender-specific. For women, they added the nourishing herbs chaste tree berry and dong quai plus six B-vitamins and named the formula Women's Renew. For men, they added the male support herbs Asian ginseng, sarsaparilla root, and saw palmetto berry plus zinc and called the formula Men's Rebuild.

Because people are increasingly concerned about the negative effects of foreign and pathogenic microorganisms in their intestines, Herbal Guard was developed, drawing upon the wisdom of Western, Native American, Chinese, and Ayurvedic herbalists. The synergistic effects of this herbal formula gently support the detoxification of your digestive system, blood, and lymph while providing nutrients to nourish cellular health. If cell health is improved, then so is your total health.

BACKGROUND INFORMATION

A leader in the field of internal cleansing, Yerba Prima sponsored a study in the 1980s to objectively validate the beneficial results reported by people who had used their program and to contribute to the scientific literature in the area of intestinal health. The study was conducted using the original formulation, Kalenite, along with the Colon Care Formula. The study was designed by Dr. Jeffrey Bland and was performed at the Linus Pauling Institute. The results of the study showed reduced numbers of pathogenic or harmful bacteria in the colon; a significant increase in absorption of water-soluble vitamins; and significant decrease in the putrefaction of undigested protein, indicating better protein absorption by the digestive tract.

Perhaps the most important discovery was that the study subjects felt better after completing the cleanse. They responded with an improved sense of well-being, lower frequency of headaches, and higher energy levels. In fact, they felt so much better that several subjects who had initially been hesitant to begin the cleansing program expressed a desire to use this cleansing program several times a year. The test results showed that the program actively worked to cleanse both the small intestine and the colon. The test subjects were ordinary people who had normal diets and bowel habits and were in good health. They did not shop in health food stores or use herbal products. No dietary changes were requested of them during the study. The study summary said that "even better results" could be expected from this program for people with chronic constipation, poor digestion, prolonged transit times, or low-fiber diets. Generally, "normal" subjects have few effects with health interventions, whereas those who have symptoms or who are ill have pronounced effects.

Yerba Prima has since upgraded the original Kalenite formula to address more current concerns about dysbiosis (see Figure 8.2)—an overgrowth of pathogenic microbes of all sorts, including bacteria, yeasts, and parasites. The improved formula is the first herbal program I know of that is designed for both complete internal cleansing and rebuilding of good digestion. Because we are exposed to numerous toxins and stresses every day, we need special assistance to maintain good health.

Ingredients of the Internal Cleansing Program

Men's Rebuild (in the men's program) contains yellow dock root, dandelion root and leaf, Asian ginseng root, ginger root, milk thistle seed, sarsaparilla root, blessed thistle herb, plantain leaf, red clover tops, saw palmetto berry, corn silk, and zinc chelate.

Women's Renew (in the women's program) contains yellow dock root, dandelion root and leaf, chaste tree berry, ginger root, milk thistle seed, dong quai root, blessed thistle herb, red clover tops, plantain leaf, corn silk, zinc chelate, folic acid, niacin, vitamin B_6, vitamin B_{12}, biotin, and pantothenic acid.

Herbal Guard (in both programs) contains triphala, elecampane root, ginger root, schisandra berry, cloves, dandelion root and leaf, cat's claw root, black walnut hull, and goldenseal root.

Here is a breakdown of the ingredients for Women's Renew, Men's Rebuild, and Herbal Guard in alphabetical order:

B-VITAMINS (FOLIC ACID, NIACIN, B_6, B_{12}, BIOTIN, PANTOTHENIC ACID)   Builds: energy, cellular health

Women's Renew contains a balanced blend of six B-vitamins to help support energy levels and cellular health during the cleansing process. These vitamins are essential for maintaining and rebuilding proper digestive and immune function, in addition to numerous other benefits of the individual B-vitamins.

BLACK WALNUT HULLS *(JUGLANS NIGRA)*   Cleanses: colon

Black walnut hulls are a traditional herb for killing and removing worms and parasites from the body. They also have antifungal properties, including specific effects against *Candida* yeast.

BLESSED THISTLE *(CNICUS BENEDICTUS)*   Cleanses: stomach, liver, gallbladder
Builds: digestion

Blessed thistle has been used for hundreds of years as one of our best mild digestive tonics. Its bitter effect improves digestion and promotes secretion of bile from the liver. Compounds contained within blessed thistle have an antimicrobial effect.

CAT'S CLAW *(UNCARIA TOMENTOSA)*   Cleanses: entire digestive tract and colon
Builds: immune system

Cat's claw, also known as "uña de gato," has been used for hundreds of years by the native people of Peru. It has strong immune-system-stimulating properties and promotes the removal of parasites. It also cleanses and heals the entire digestive tract, which helps with many stomach and colon disorders via its anti-inflammatory and antioxidant properties.

Chaste tree berry (*Vitex agnus-castus*)   Builds: proper hormonal function

Chaste tree berry is a building and balancing herb for women. It is used in European herbalism as a tonic and normalizer for the female reproductive system because it helps normalize the activity of female sex hormones. This property gives chaste tree berry a wide range of uses, especially in menopause and with menstrual irregularities. Studies in Europe have shown that over time, this herb helps to reduce discomfort related to PMS (premenstrual syndrome).

Cloves (*Syzygium aromaticum*)   Cleanses: colon (anti-parasitic), lungs
Builds: digestion

Cloves contain a volatile oil that gives them warming, carminative properties in the stomach and digestive system, which helps to reduce flatulence. It is another synergistic ingredient in this formula that helps remove worms and parasites from the colon. It is a mild stimulant with expectorant and lung-clearing properties.

Corn silk (*Zea mays*)   Cleanses: kidneys and urinary system

Corn silk has been used for hundreds of years, primarily as a soothing diuretic for the kidneys. It helps reduce inflammation in the urinary system and has a mild cleansing effect on the liver.

DANDELION LEAF AND ROOT *(TARAXACUM OFFICINALE)*
Cleanses: liver, gallbladder, kidneys, blood, skin
Builds: liver and kidney health, nutritive for the entire body

This common weed is used as both food and medicine. We recognize it as an herb for its safe, nutritive, diuretic effect on the kidneys (it is high in potassium) and its ability to stimulate the release of bile and the contraction of the gallbladder, which promotes better bowel movements. David Hoffmann, in *Holistic Herbal,* says, "This herb is a most valuable general tonic and perhaps the best widely applicable diuretic and liver tonic."[1] Dandelion has been used for hundreds of years in Europe, the Middle East, China, and India. The first written reference to dandelion as a medicine was from Arabic physicians of the tenth and eleventh centuries. Because dandelion contains polysaccharides, such as inulin, it may provide immune support. It is also known to have anti-inflammatory properties. If dandelion were not such a common plant, and such a pest to the gardener and the grower of manicured lawns, it would probably be hailed as a miracle herb.

As a food, dandelion leaves can be eaten like a vegetable. Tender young leaves add a spark to any salad, and the older, larger leaves are nice to add to sautéed greens for a rich flavor. They are high in vitamins. The roots when roasted have been savored as a coffee substitute.

DONG QUAI ROOT *(ANGELICA SINENSIS)*   Cleanses: blood
Protects: circulatory system, liver
Builds: blood, reproductive system

Dong quai is widely used in Asia, and is considered the premier women's tonic herb. It is used to build the blood and improve circulation. Its other major function is to tone a woman's reproductive system. For these reasons, it is widely used throughout the reproductive years as well as during menopause.

Dong quai has secondary benefits of protecting the liver, providing mild laxative effects in cases of dry intestines from deficient blood, and contributing antimicrobial properties against many types of bacteria.

ELECAMPANE ROOT (*INULA HELENIUM*)   Cleanses: respiratory system, colon (antiparasitic)
Builds: digestion, general tonic herb

Elecampane root is one of the best antiparasitic herbs. It helps eliminate parasites such as giardia, amebic infections, and pinworms. Even though it is strong, it is safe to use over a long period of time. Traditionally it has been used for the respiratory system, helping to soothe the mucous membranes while clearing and strengthening the lungs and bronchial system. It has mild carminative properties, like ginger and cloves, that soothe digestive upset. Its mild bitter properties improve digestion.

GINGER ROOT (*ZINGIBER OFFICINALE*)   Cleanses: stomach, small intestine, circulatory system, liver
Builds: digestion, stomach, colon, circulatory system

Ginger is carminative. Carminative herbs contain essential oils and other constituents that calm the digestive system through their warming, antispasmodic, and anti-inflammatory actions. Cleansing puts stress on the digestive system. Ginger and cloves help to neutralize this stress. Through its anti-inflammatory properties, ginger reduces gas, indigestion, and nausea and has mild pain-relieving effects. It is helpful for motion sickness, and studies show that it is at least as effective as prescription drugs now used for the same purpose without the possible side effects.

Ginger has been used for thousands of years in the Chinese, Ayurvedic, and Western healing traditions, and it tastes good in food or as a tea that stimulates metabolism. Other beneficial effects include increased bile secretion, antioxidant protection for the liver, antibacterial properties, antiparasitic properties (helps eliminate worms), heart protection by lowering cholesterol and inhibiting platelet aggregation, normalization of bowel function, and restoration of colon tone.

GOLDENSEAL ROOT EXTRACT *(HYDRASTIS CANADENSIS)*
Cleanses: digestive system, lungs, reproductive system
Builds: health of mucous membranes, stomach
Goldenseal is widely used among Native Americans, who taught the use of this herb to European settlers. It is one of the best tonic herbs when used in small quantities, as in this formula. In large amounts, it is antimicrobial for mucous membranes of the digestive, respiratory, and reproductive systems. Its bitter quality promotes bile production, improves digestion, and encourages proper bowel movements. Goldenseal has anti-inflammatory, antibacterial, and antiparasitic properties and is mildly stimulating to the immune system.

MILK THISTLE SEED *(SILYBUM MARIANUM)* Cleanses: liver, kidneys, blood, skin
Builds: digestion
Milk thistle seed is a mild digestive bitter used in treating skin disorders for its effect on cleansing the blood.

Used since antiquity for digestive and liver complaints, it increases secretion and flow of bile. It gently promotes liver cleansing, but its primary actions go beyond that as one of the strongest liver herbs known. It both protects the liver with its antioxidant properties and rebuilds by supporting RNA synthesis.

The toxins that the liver neutralizes come from within us as well as from the outside world. During the cleansing process, the liver has extra work to do as toxins are released from tissues of the body into the blood and lymph. Milk thistle seed extract protects the liver cells as they neutralize toxins, bind to them, and dump them into the colon for elimination from the body. At the same time, it works to rebuild damaged liver tissue.

The primary activity of this herb is due to compounds in the seeds known as silymarin, a group of flavolignan (a large class of substances found in plants that have healing properties) compounds that have been studied extensively for the past few decades, primarily in Europe. Silymarin has been used successfully to treat patients who have chronic hepatitis and cirrhosis; it is active against the hepatitis B virus, and it lowers fat deposits in the liver in animals.

Historical use of milk thistle as a liver herb dates back to the first century. Pliny the Elder, a Roman naturalist, tells us that the juice of the plant mixed with honey is excellent for "carrying off bile." (Bile is a concentrated liver product that is excreted from the gallbladder in response to dietary fats in the small intestines.)

Recently, European doctors have found that they can save the lives of most people who would have died from mistakenly eating the poisonous *Amanita phalloides* mushroom ("death cap"). They do this by intravenous drip injection of a pure extract of milk thistle seed called Silibinin within 48 hours of exposure. Prior to this discovery, about 25 percent of the unfortunate mushroom hunters died from hemorrhagic necrosis of the liver, or they had to undergo liver transplant surgery with subsequent immunosuppressive therapy for the rest of their lives to help them tolerate the transplant organ.

Because of its effect on cleansing the blood, milk thistle is also used for treating skin disorders.

PLANTAIN LEAF *(PLANTAGO MAJOR* OR *PLANTAGO LANCEO-LATA)*   Cleanses: kidneys and urinary system, respiratory system, colon

Plantain leaf is a soothing herb with mild diuretic, expectorant, and digestion-enhancing properties. It is an excellent supportive- herb for the cleansing process. Plantain contains mucilage, which provides soothing action and helps heal inflamed tissue in the colon and rectum. Plantain leaf juice and syrups have been used in Europe to reduce symptoms of bronchitis and respiratory problems. It has mild liver-cleansing, bowel-regulating, and antimicrobial properties.

RED CLOVER TOPS *(TRIFOLIUM PRATENSE)*   Cleanses: blood, liver, lymphatic system
Builds: blood; balances hormones

Red clover has been an agricultural crop for animals for thousands of years because of its high nutrient content. It has also been used in healing traditions around the world, primarily as a mild cleansing and protecting herb. Recent research shows that red clover has particular value for women's health. It is a rich source of isoflavone compounds, which help to balance hormone levels, especially during menopause.

SARSAPARILLA ROOT *(SMILAX SPP.)*   Cleanses: blood
Protects: liver, colon
Builds: energy levels, blood

Sarsaparilla root is not only an ingredient in soft drinks. It is a tonic and a building herb used in many cultures around the world for its gentle strengthening properties. More recently, it has been widely used by athletes to support the muscle-building and strengthening process.

Traditionally, sarsaparilla root has been used to treat rheumatism and skin conditions in both Europe and Asia. It works through the liver and kidneys to cleanse and build the blood. In addition, it contributes mild anti-inflammatory properties.

SAW PALMETTO BERRY *(SERENOA REPENS)*   Protects: prostate
Builds: general nutritional support

Saw palmetto berry helps strengthen the male reproductive system. It is best known for its ability to protect and support proper functioning of the prostate gland. This has been proven in numerous double-blind studies in Europe, even compared with prescription drugs used to treat benign prostatic hypertrophy. Traditionally, saw palmetto berry has been used by Native Americans as a nutritive tonic.

SCHISANDRA BERRY *(SCHISANDRA CHINENSIS)*   Cleanses: liver
Builds: liver, energy, digestion, adrenal glands

In your liver, the adaptogen schisandra offers strong liver protection; it is an antioxidant that promotes the repair of damaged liver tissue. It promotes better digestion, builds kidney function, and normalizes stomach acidity. Through its mild stimulating effect on the central nervous system, it promotes energy gently while increasing stamina and endurance.

Studies have shown that schisandra has the ability to quicken reflexes and improve a person's ability to concentrate.

ASIAN GINSENG ROOT *(PANAX GINSENG)*   Protects: immune system
Builds: adrenal glands, energy levels

Asian ginseng root has been used as an adaptogen (an herb that helps the body and mind adapt to stress) in China for more than 2,000 years. Traditional Chinese medicine calls Asian ginseng a warming tonic that provides both mental/emotional support and strengthening of physical energy. Recent scientific research has shown that it helps reduce fatigue, supports the immune system, and helps maintain healthy blood sugar levels. Asian ginseng is a deep energy builder but not a stimulant like caffeine. It is slightly stronger than either Siberian or American ginseng and supports male energy during the internal cleansing process.

TRIPHALA (A COMBINATION *PHYLLANTHUS EMBLICA, TERMINALIA BALLERICA,* AND *TERMINALIA CHEBULA)*   Cleanses: stomach, small intestine, colon, respiratory system
Builds: stomach, small intestine, colon, overall digestion

This herb combination comes to us from Ayurveda, the ancient East Indian tradition of healing. Traditionally, triphala has been used as a bowel normalizer for constipation or diarrhea and to improve the tone of the colon through the astringent properties of tannins. Triphala helps purify the blood through its actions against bacteria, yeast, fungi, parasites, and worms. It promotes normal appetite and good digestion and improves the absorption of B-vitamins. Like ginseng in Asia, triphala is used as an adaptogen and a rejuvenating food in the Ayurvedic system of health care. It is of special value both as a regulator of elimination and a revitalizer of the entire body.

Yellow dock root *(Rumex crispus)* Cleanses: liver, gallbladder, colon, blood, lymph, respiratory system, skin
Builds: liver, blood, digestive system

Yellow dock root supports the function of the liver and gall bladder by promoting bile secretion and flow, which indirectly supports the colon with a gentle laxative action. Throughout history, bitters such as yellow dock root have been used to stimulate appetite and digestion. (Bitters are herbs that activate gastric secretion of hydrochloric acid and other digestive enzymes such as bile.) Another historical use of this herb, which goes back thousands of years, is for cleansing. Yellow dock root was widely used by almost 20 Native American tribes. Through its antibacterial properties, it improves skin condition. It is also high in iron and promotes better use of iron in the body. Over time, it has a gentle effect that helps promote regular elimination.

Prima Cleanse

To complement the herbal activity of Herbal Guard, Women's Renew, and Men's Rebuild, Yerba Prima developed a high-fiber formula called Prima Cleanse as an essential part of the cleansing program. (See chapters 3 and 7 for information on the importance of dietary fiber.) Mixed fiber products produce the best anticancer effects. This formula is made from a variety of fiber sources, plus other protective nutrients, and is designed to perform the following functions:

- absorb the toxins that are being released by the body into the colon (Animal studies indicate that various drugs, chemicals, and food additives are highly toxic when fed to rats and mice in conjunction with a purified, low-fiber diet; when fed diets high in dietary fiber, the same doses have no deleterious effects.)
- speed the toxic-laden feces out of the body rapidly and regularly
- promote stools that are larger, softer, and easier to evacuate
- reduce pressure in the colon and lessen the risk of diverticulosis, hemorrhoids, and other colon disorders
- help build the population of friendly bacteria in the intestines, thus encouraging a strong and toxin-free system
- provide "food" to the colon's friendly bacteria to enhance the production of B-vitamins, mammalian lignans, and SCFAs (short-chain fatty acids), which are a by-product of friendly intestinal bacteria and act as a nutrient source for cells lining the intestinal tract (thus protecting against cancer and helping to maintain the integrity of the colon lining)
- increase absorption of nutrients across the bowel wall
- decrease the risk of colon, breast, and prostate cancer
- decrease the risk of heart disease
- soothe and protect the intestinal lining during the cleansing process

The ingredients in Prima Cleanse work together to achieve optimal benefits (see pages 170–173 for usage). Prima Cleanse capsules (in both the Women's and Men's programs) contain the following fibers and colon-nourishing supplements: psyllium husks, aloe vera gel, ginger root, Great Plains Bentonite, senna leaf, calcium carbonate, FOS Probiotic Growth Complex (fructo-oligosaccharides), magnesium oxide, soy fiber, acacia gum, oat bran, and apple pectin extract.

The following is a breakdown of the ingredients in Prima Cleanse in alphabetical order:

ACACIA GUM   Builds: intestinal tract by feeding healthy bacteria and intestinal cells

Acacia gum is a concentrated source of soluble fiber. Unlike most soluble fibers, it does not form thick solutions when mixed with water. Acacia gum is totally broken down as a food source for beneficial intestinal bacteria, such as bifs and other friendly bacteria increasing their numbers in your colon. With the increase in bacterial mass, it also slightly increases the bulk material in the colon. However, it does not improve transit time like psyllium husks and soy fiber do.

Acacia gum has been shown to slightly reduce elevated cholesterol levels. Its effect is not as strong as that of psyllium husks, oat bran, or pectin. In human trials, the addition of acacia gum to a measured glucose (sugar) dose resulted in significant reduction of sugar and insulin in the blood when taken at the same time. It acts as a demulcent, or soothing substance, for the lining of the intestinal tract. It is widely used in foods such as beverages, salad dressings, and sauces as a carrier for flavors and as a stabilizer. Like FOSs, but to a lesser extent, acacia gum protects colon cells against cancer by increasing their depth; the cells actually become deeper, thus improving the health of the bowel. (Cells are supposed to be deep; when they are not, it is a sign of cancer.)

ALOE VERA   Protects: soothes and heals the lining of the stomach, small intestine, and colon
Builds: digestive health, immune system health

Aloe vera is known as "the burn plant" because so many people keep an aloe vera plant growing in the kitchen to apply to the skin in case of burns. Similarly, aloe vera provides soothing and healing properties internally throughout the digestive system. During an active cleansing process, digestion can be stressed in some people, and aloe vera works with ginger root and other soothing herbs in the program to provide balance. (See more detailed information about aloe vera on pages 214–218.)

CALCIUM CARBONATE   Cleanses: colon
Builds: bones, circulatory system; holds cells together

Colon cancer is the second most common cancer in women and the third most common in men. Animals and people who eat a high-fat, low-fiber diet get colon cancer more often. When animals are injected with carcinogenic substances, those fed high-fat diets have a higher incidence of cancer than those fed low-fat diets. Calcium is protective against colon cancer. It works through several different modes of action. Supplementing dietary calcium at about 1.5 times the Recommended Dietary Allowance (for a total of 1,500 milligrams/day) restores the cells of your colon wall to a more normal and quiet equilibrium, reducing the over-proliferation that occurs with cancer growth. And calcium that is not absorbed by the small intestine enters the colon and binds with rancid fats and excess bile acids to form harmless insoluble soaps. The protective properties of calcium complement the protective properties of insoluble fiber.

High phosphate levels in the diet, from soda and carbonated beverages, will cause phosphate to bind with calcium and reduce its ability to remove rancid fats, toxins, and excess bile acids from the colon.

FOS Probiotic Growth Complex (also known as fructo-oligosaccharides)   Cleanses: colon
Builds: colon cells, friendly intestinal bacteria

Fructo-oligosaccharides (FOSs) are naturally occurring complex sugars that have beneficial effects when included in your diet. They can be found in rye, banana, onion, garlic, burdock, asparagus, chicory root, and Jerusalem artichoke. Judging from usual eating habits, it may be difficult to ingest the recommended daily doses of FOSs from foods. Most animal and human diets are deficient in FOSs.

In addition, most modern people engage in activities that cause damage to their intestines: overconsumption of alcohol; eating raw eggs, fish, and seafood that may produce bacterial infections; use of aspirin and other painkillers; use of antibiotics; and poor diet. Even the water we drink may prove harmful (see chapter 6).

Every year, more than 35 million pounds of antibiotics are consumed by humans, livestock, and poultry in the United States. You may unknowingly consume secondhand antibiotics hidden in meat, poultry, and dairy products unless you eat organic animal products raised without the use of antibiotics. The overall effect of our antibiotic habit has been not only the destruction of helpful bacteria in the intestines but also the establishment of harmful strains of bacteria that antibiotics can no longer kill.

Over the last 30 years of antibiotic use, strains of bacteria have mutated to become antibiotic-resistant for almost every known bacterial disease. In 1972, 13,300 hospital patients died of infections that resisted every drug their doctor tried, and in 1993 the number grew to 70,000. Dr. Bill Jarvis of the Centers for Disease Control and Prevention in Atlanta, Georgia, said, "[Resistance to antibiotics] is probably the number-one public health issue."

Unless you eat a significant quantity of foods high in FOSs, you would benefit from the addition of FOS products to your daily regimen such as Colon Care Formula from Yerba Prima or Ultra Flora Plus and Probioplex Intensive Care from Metagenics (see appendix 1 for ordering information). Extensive animal and human studies have established the safety and efficacy of FOSs. It is now used as an ingredient in more than 500 food products in Japan. In studies done with FOSs, stool markers (laboratory stool tests) dropped down to less healthy levels when FOSs were withdrawn from the diet. Health contributions of FOSs arise from its unique fermentation characteristics:

- FOSs increase the population of bifidobacteria (bifs) and lactobacilli in your colon even without adding probiotic cultures to your diet. The FOS-nourished bifs decrease stool pH, thus inhibiting the growth of undesirable organisms and stimulating your gut's immune system, perhaps due to an increased production of SCFAs. By suppressing the activity of undesirable putrefactive bacteria, such as *E. coli, Salmonella,* and *Clostridium perfringens,* bifs reduce the formation of their toxic fermentation products. This in turn protects your liver function by reducing levels of toxic bowel metabolites. Your liver is saved from having to process these harmful by-products of a low-fiber, high-fat diet and poor digestion.

- People with diarrhea and soft, loose stools found that their stools became firmer and that constipation was prevented through production of SCFAs, which stimulate bowel motility (peristalsis) and increase fecal moisture and osmotic pressure.

- Sustained intake of FOSs among the Japanese in the mid-1980s resulted in significant reductions in cholesterol and triglyceride levels, just like adding additional fiber. Fiber and FOSs had a synergistic effect. FOSs also caused a reduction of blood pressure; the more bifs present, the lower the diastolic blood pressure (the bottom number, which indicates the pressure in your heart).

- FOSs have an anticancer effect due to immunity enhancements by the cells, cell wall components, and extracellular components of bifidobacteria.

- FOSs support production of vitamins B_1, B_2, B_3, B_6, and B_{12} and folic acid. These are all part of the B-complex vitamins, which support your brain, nervous system, digestion, and energy production.

FRUIT PECTIN   Cleanses: intestinal tract, circulatory system (lower cholesterol and blood glucose)
Builds: colon health

Pectin is a soluble fiber that is found in all fruits and vegetables but especially in apples and citrus fruit. It has a number of beneficial properties in the body. It lowers elevated cholesterol levels, as do many soluble fibers. However, other properties are more important.

Pectin is almost entirely fermented by intestinal bacteria, which means that it is used as a food source by the "good guys" in your intestines. As you have previously read, these friendly bacteria synthesize B-vitamins, acidify the colon, produce SCFAs, protect the colon, and keep harmful bacteria and yeasts in check.

Consumed with meals, pectin increases the excretion of fecal fat, neutral steroids, and fecal bile acids. By increasing the excretion of fecal neutral steroids, it helps reduce your risk of sex-hormone-related cancers. Remember that old adage, "An apple a day keeps the doctor away." Apples are high in pectin, ridding your body of excess cancer-stimulating hormones.

The addition of pectin to a drink or meal significantly reduces blood glucose response. Pectin would be a helpful addition to the diets of people with diabetes. However, the benefit depends on the presence of pectin in the intestine during the sugar stress. The sugar-stabilizing effect is also felt by people who do not have diabetes; blood sugar swings and drastic changes in mood and energy are diminished.

The addition of pectin to the diet, unlike other fiber sources such as wheat bran, does not decrease the level of minerals (e.g., calcium, magnesium, zinc, and copper) in the blood. However, iron levels were decreased by pectin in some but not all human studies.

Pectin is also known to pick up heavy metals as it goes through the digestive tract. Russian research showed that pectin and pectin-containing foods increased the excretion of lead, mercury, manganese, and beryllium from the gastrointestinal tract. It also protected animals and people from lead poisoning when taken before and during exposure to lead.

GINGER ROOT *(ZINGIBER OFFICINALE)*   Ginger root is a warming, protective digestive herb.

GREAT PLAINS BENTONITE   Cleanses: stomach, small intestines and colon
This special, activated form of bentonite is added to the formula for its strong detoxifying properties. Whereas fiber ingredients swell and absorb toxins and waste material as they pass through the digestive system and colon, bentonite adsorbs toxins through chemical attraction and pulls them out of the body.

OAT BRAN   Cleanses: colon
Builds: health of circulatory system; lowers elevated cholesterol and triglyceride levels; high in nutrients for whole body
Dozens of studies have consistently shown that oat bran consumption significantly reduces elevated cholesterol and triglyceride levels. The soluble-fiber portion of oat bran is believed to be responsible for this benefit. About half of the fiber in oat bran is soluble fiber. In this way, the humble oat can help reduce the risk of heart diseases while providing nutrition.
Oat bran should not be confused with fiber from the hull of the oat, sometimes called oat fiber. The hull is removed before oats are used for human food, and it is entirely insoluble fiber. It does not have the cholesterol-lowering properties

of oat bran, and some unscrupulous companies sell it because it costs less than oat bran.

PSYLLIUM SEED HUSKS   Cleanses: intestinal tract
Protects: colon and circulatory systems (lowers cholesterol)
Builds: colon cells

Psyllium was first introduced as a commercial product in the United States not by health food stores but by the Kellogg brothers, according to the director of research at Kellogg's. John Harvey Kellogg found psyllium on a trip to Sicily and introduced it at the Battle Creek Sanitarium. Beginning in the 1920s, it was sold at the sanitarium under the name Psylla. After the sanitarium folded, psyllium was forgotten by Kellogg's until the late 1980s. At that time, Kellogg's scientists were seeing research that soluble fiber helped lower cholesterol levels and reduce the risk of heart disease. Kellogg's had found great sales success with their educational campaign telling people how fiber could reduce the risk of cancer and saw the possibility for similar success with a soluble-fiber cereal. So Kellogg's scientists tested 100 different sources of soluble fibers and decided that psyllium was the best of all. Psyllium husk is highly concentrated in its activity and retains its effectiveness even after processing into a breakfast cereal. But Kellogg's psyllium-based cereals have not met sales expectations in the United States, and the Heartwise brand was discontinued. However, Kellogg's has a better-selling psyllium cereal in Australia being marketed for heart health.

For health and cleansing, psyllium husk is the best choice. However, other fiber sources have important benefits. Psyllium is the most exciting because of its broad range of cleansing actions in the body. It has the properties of both soluble and insoluble fibers. In general, insoluble fibers add bulk and attract water into your bowel, whereas soluble fibers are responsible for the other heart-healthy, cancer-protective, bacteria-building properties. Psyllium fiber both adds bulk, acting as a gentle broom for your intestinal lining, and lowers cholesterol levels to protect your cardiovascular system against heart attacks.

No cleansing program can be successful without removing toxins from the colon, and studies have shown that no fiber is as powerful as psyllium husks for trapping and removing toxins. Imagine a sponge that expands 40 to 70 times its original size, with expanded scrubbing power. That gives you a picture of the power of psyllium. Psyllium husks form a soft, bulky mass that gently scrubs the walls of the intestines as it moves through your digestive tract. At the same time, it traps toxins and excess cholesterol and flushes them out of your body.

Psyllium contributes to the cleansing process in a multitude of ways. In addition to scrubbing the colon walls and removing toxins, it promotes a shorter transit time. This means that the body's waste material spends less time in your colon and has less contact with the mucosa of your colon.

Psyllium husks strengthen the integrity of the intestinal lining, reducing the chance of bacteria and intestinal toxins penetrating through the wall and into your bloodstream. Animal studies have shown that adding fiber to a liquid diet reduces the amount of bacteria crossing the intestinal wall and getting into the circulation by almost 90 percent. This may be accomplished through the nourishment SCFAs provide to the cells that line the intestines. As a soluble fiber, psyllium husks promote the growth of friendly bacteria in the colon. Friendly bacteria support the cleansing process and help restore normal bowel function.

SENNA LEAF   Cleanses: colon

Senna leaf has been used around the world for hundreds of years as a reliable stimulator of bowel activity. Senna was known primarily in the Middle East until around the time of the Crusades, when it was introduced to Europeans. Native American tribes have also used plants related to senna for similar purposes. A small amount of senna leaf extract in Prima Cleanse helps to ensure the removal of waste material and cleansing of the colon during the program. It is especially valuable for people who have a slow metabolism or sluggish bowel activity.

SOY FIBER   Cleanses: colon
Builds: healthy bacteria

Soy is a concentrated source of insoluble dietary fiber, which helps to promote regular, healthy bowel movements. Insoluble fiber helps speed transit time so toxins do not stay so long in the body and acts as a stimulator for healthy bacteria growth in the colon. Yerba Prima uses the most active portion of the soybean for its cleansing benefits. Soy fiber exerts a protective effect in the colon through its bulking activity.

USAGE INSTRUCTIONS

Although each person's needs will vary, in this section I provide general guidelines for following a detoxification program with the Yerba Prima Herb and Fiber Cleansing Program.

Recommended Amounts Per Serving for Yerba Prima Cleanse

Women

Time Period	Prima Cleanse	Herbal Guard	Women's Renew
First evening	3		
Days 2 and 3	3	1	1
2 to 8 weeks— gentler	3	1	1
2 to 8 weeks— stronger	5	2	2

Men

Time Period	Prima Cleanse	Herbal Guard	Men's Rebuild
First evening	3		
Days 2 and 3	3	1	1
2 to 8 weeks— gentler	3	1	1
2 to 8 weeks— stronger	5	2	2

Consult your health-care practitioner before beginning any detoxification program. If problems arise, stop using the products and consult with your health-care practitioner. Pregnant and lactating women should not engage in detoxification but instead would benefit from using a fiber supplement only.

These instructions apply to both the Women's Renew and the Men's Rebuild Cleansing Programs. You can jump-start the cleansing process by taking 3 Prima Cleanse capsules the evening of the first day with a minimum of 8 ounces of pure water. For the next 2 days, take 3 Prima Cleanse, 1 Herbal Guard, and 1 Women's Renew or Men's

Rebuild twice a day, morning and evening, with at least 8 ounces of pure water.

On the fourth day, evaluate whether your body is already having a strong response to the cleansing herbs and fiber. If you are having more frequent or much larger bowel movements than normal for you, then the cleanse is working and you should continue at this gentle level for at least 2 weeks and up to 2 months. If the cleansing action is too strong at any time, reduce the number of Prima Cleanse capsules you are taking or switch to Yerba Prima's milder Colon Care Formula or Caps fiber supplement to adjust the cleansing action to suit your body's needs.

If by the fourth day you are not having larger or more frequent bowel movements, increase your dosage to 5 Prima Cleanse, 2 Herbal Guard, and 2 Women's Renew or Men's Rebuild twice a day, morning and evening, with at least 8 ounces of pure water. You can continue at this level for at least 2 weeks and up to 2 months. Again, if the cleansing action becomes too strong at any time, moderate it by reducing the number of Prima Cleanse capsules you take or switching the fiber supplement to Yerba Prima's Colon Care Formula or Caps.

A rule of thumb is to try to keep the cleansing activity in your body at a level that produces two to three regular, easy, non-urgent bowel movements per day. When you finish the cleansing program, you may find that regular use of a fiber product such as Colon Care Formula or Caps helps maintain good digestive health. This would be especially true for people who tend to eat a low-fiber diet.

You will benefit from this cleansing program with almost any kind of diet. However, you will increase your benefits significantly by following these daily dietary guidelines:

- eat five servings of fruits and vegetables
- reduce or eliminate intake of hydrogenated, partially hydrogenated, and fractionated oils; animal fats; and sugary foods
- drink sufficient pure water for your body weight to aid detoxification

Keeping a diary to chart your progress will help you appreciate the necessity and benefit of engaging in regular detoxification programs. The Bowel Movement Progress Chart (page 194) can assist your progress toward vibrant good health.

CHAPTER 10

THERAPEUTIC FOOD POWDERS FOR CLEANSING

Cleansing programs that use therapeutic food powders spare protein loss and provide specific nutrition for the support and repair of organ systems during detoxification. Dr. Jeffrey Bland has developed a line of therapeutic food powders that are effective at cleansing the body and supporting your inherent ability to heal. The therapeutic foods are tasty and easy to use. I personally use these products almost daily, and for regular cleansing programs several times per year. It's easy to get good nutrition with this Ultra line of products. They are reasonably priced, and they beat chopping, cooking, and cleaning up after yourself when you have limited time. Many of my patients and clients, as do I, choose to have an Ultra drink for breakfast. Because the food powders are made of small food molecules, they are easy to digest and absorb when you are in a rush to eat before or during your workday. The cleansing Ultra products—Ultra Clear, Ultra Clear Plus, Ultra Clear Sustain, Ultra InflamX, and Ultra

GlycemX—are available only through offices of licensed health-care practitioners. Cleansing programs using these products must be performed in conjunction with a health-care practitioner who can determine the specifics regarding quantity, dosage, frequency, length of the cleanse, and the most appropriate food powder to use.

Dr. Bland and a group of registered dietitians, scientists, and medical doctors conducted studies using these products. In order to assess the need for cleansing and chart the progress of the subjects tested, several tools were used, including the Metabolic Screening Questionnaire (MSQ) in chapter 8 and a liver function test called the Functional Liver Detoxification Profile (FLDP), which measured the breakdown products of caffeine and sodium benzoate in saliva and urine. The FLDP measures the detoxification processes of the liver. These tests differ from the normal liver blood tests in that the FLDP measures the ability of the liver to do its job, whereas normal blood tests measure the enzymes from dying (necrosing) liver tissue.

The FLDP is a measure of how your body detoxifies commonly used liver stressors: caffeine, acetaminophen, and aspirin. Caffeine is converted into a benign substance through a process in the liver called the "phase I cytochrome P450 mixed oxidase pathway." Aspirin and acetaminophen are metabolized through both the "phase I and phase II pathways." Phase I detoxification is stimulated through exposure to xenobiotics, steroids, toxics produced inside the body, alcohol, and chemical substances. If you are the kind of person who has a marked reaction to caffeine that lasts for hours and interferes with your ability to sleep even though you may have had it early in the day, then you probably have suppressed phase I detoxification in your liver.

(Remember Tom Latimer in chapter 5? His phase I detoxification was suppressed by the medication Tagamet.) Phase I detoxification converts toxics and normal chemical substances such as hormones into intermediary metabolites; these are often more dangerous and carcinogenic than the chemicals to which a person was initially exposed. That is why you need a well-functioning phase II: to complete the job of phase I and make those toxic intermediary metabolites into benign end-products that can be safely eliminated from your body, primarily through secretion into your blood and subsequent excretion in urine through your kidneys, but also through secretion into the bile and subsequent excretion in the feces.

Have you or someone you know experienced a "cleansing reaction" when you were attempting to detoxify your body? What's happening in this situation is that phase I detoxification has been stimulated, or upregulated, without having the support of ample nutrients to complete the process through phase II into harmless products. The intermediary metabolites instead re-enter your bloodstream and wreak havoc among your many cells and body systems. If you are a "canary" with multiple food and chemical sensitivities who is bothered by the smell of perfume and car fumes, especially diesel exhaust (perfumes are often derivatives of petroleum), you probably have too little phase II conjugates to detoxify the intermediary metabolites produced by phase I in your liver.

What Dr. Bland's team of researchers found was amazing. In a study of normal, nondiseased, but unwell people, published in the *Journal of Applied Nutrition*,[1] doctors Bland and Bralley found that the chronic symptoms in the group that was using Ultra Clear were much lower in intensity, duration, and frequency than among those on the placebo diet. The greatest improvements occurred with "tired eyes" and "pain behind the eyes," headaches, gastrointestinal disturbances, morning pain and stiffness, and chronic respiratory complaints. The therapeutic food group's objective laboratory test results improved more than the placebo diet group. The MSQ scores for the test diet group lowered significantly; scores for the placebo group did not. Both phases of liver detoxification for the test group worked better; the placebo group did not improve significantly. The study report states: "These data suggest a relationship between improved liver detoxification and decreased chronic symptoms and health complaints in non-diseased people." The therapeutic food group gained better health in only 21 days.

AN EFFECTIVE CLEANSING PROGRAM FOR OVERCOMING CHRONIC FATIGUE

Chronic Fatigue Immunodeficiency Syndrome (CFIDS) is thought to be caused by a viral agent. A study entitled, "Entero-hepatic resuscitation program for CFIDS" by Doctor Rigden shows that, for some, the signs and symptoms of CFIDS can be relieved by supporting liver detoxification.[2] Perhaps you don't fit the Center for Disease Control's criteria for CFIDS, but chances are that you feel drained sometimes. Maybe that second wind just won't seem to kick in even with your usual remedies and stimulants. Fatigue is the most common symptom that patients report to their doctor.

Doctor Rigden documented the health improvements in thirty patients who fulfilled the Center for Disease Control's criteria for CFIDS. The average time these subjects had suffered with CFIDS symptoms before participating in this study was 3 years, and they had all tried many other therapies to regain their health before trying Dr. Bland's therapeutic food, Ultra Clear. After only 7 days of following the nutritional intervention program based on Ultra Clear, the test subjects showed marked improvement in eye, respiratory, central nervous system, and musculoskeletal symptoms. Whereas the Metabolic Screening Questionnaire mean score for the nondiseased people was 44, the average score among the CFIDS participants was 173. That score dropped in half after only 1 month of nutritional intervention. The most significant reduction of symptoms was associated with improvements in vision-related problems (tired eyes and inability to read for any length of time). Other improvements included a reduction of headaches, improvements in respiratory function, reduced sinusitis and congestion, and improvements in central nervous system function.

One participant, who had been unable to work for a year, was back at work and functioning well with her family responsibilities after the nutritional intervention program. Another participant was an accountant who, due to the symptoms of CFIDS, had become unable to work with numbers. After the cleansing program, which reduced her symptoms by more than 50 percent, she was able to return to work. The clinical improvement in the symptoms and abnormalities found in the immune systems of people with CFIDS were closely related to improved activity of both phase I and II of liver detoxification in functional lab tests. They enjoyed these beneficial results from doing cleansing programs using the Ultra Clear products under the supervision of a health-care practitioner.

Although the Ultra Clear intervention proved ineffective and/or poorly tolerated by a subgroup of Chronic Fatigue Immunodeficiency Syndrome (CFIDS) patients, most patients benefited from the program. Five of those patients with a higher ratio of phase I to phase II liver detoxification entered the Ultra Clear Plus study and had a significant reduction of symptoms compared to others in the study with lower ratios. Of the 14 people in the study, none had an increase or worsening of symptoms and most reported a decrease in symptoms from 11 to 64 percent as monitored by the Metabolic Screening Questionnaire).[3]

Dr. Jeffrey Bland and his team evaluated the effectiveness of the therapeutic food supplement Ultra Clear Sustain (UCS) for detoxification versus a hypoallergenic, calorie-controlled diet alone in the management of chronically ill patients. There were 106 patients chosen for the study. The eighty-four patients in the experimental group who consumed the UCS had a 52 percent reduction in symptoms over 10 weeks using the Metabolic Screening Questionnaire (MSQ). The twenty-two patients on the control diet had only a 22 percent reduction of symptoms. In the group that used UCS, symptoms reduced and the Functional Liver Detoxification Profile (FLDP) showed normalization of both phases of liver detoxification. Enhanced nutrient absorption was implied by positive results in bowel function tests.

The patients in this study were free of serious disease. However, they suffered with fatigue, muscle and joint pain, chronic gastrointestinal problems, headaches, sleep disturbances, and cognitive impairment (which the patients often described as "brain fog") of at least one year's duration (average 2.4 years). Patients in both groups were placed on food-elimination diets to reduce their intake of the most common allergens: dairy products, gluten-containing grains, and citrus fruits. They were also asked to avoid red meat, pork, veal, and all products containing alcohol and caffeine, including over-the-counter medications.

Symptoms that improved most rapidly were those related to energy/activity, digestive functions, mood/mind/emotions, sleep, and muscle pain. Additional symptoms that improved were those related to eye pain when reading, headaches, and skin problems. In a subgroup of the therapeutic food patients who had gastrointestinal disturbances, symptoms such as flatulence, bloating, alternating constipation and diarrhea, and intestinal pain after eating were reduced after intervention. Although the control group on the food program alone showed improvement in the MSQ, no significant changes were measured in their objective lab tests.

It becomes obvious from these studies that the best way to treat your body during a cleanse is to give it nourishing, easy-to-digest foods or food powders to enhance your body's ability to heal. There are many food powders on the market. To make sure you are investing in a product that supports your health, it is best to read the ingredient list carefully. If the product has anything artificial in it, I would recommend finding another product. The same goes for sugar (sucrose, dextrose), NutraSweet (aspartame), Sweet 'n Low (saccharine), and other sweeteners like Splenda. A food powder to avoid is the popular Ultra Slim Fast that is sold in many supermarkets. It has been shown to help people lose weight, but most of the weight lost is lean weight from muscles, organs, and glands, not fat. This compromises both your health and longevity and works against your liver's ability to cleanse toxins from your body.

Chronic Fatigue Immunodeficiency Syndrome Questionnaire

1. I have experienced easy fatigability that has lasted at least 6 months.
2. A physician has evaluated me and ruled out any physical or psychiatric diseases that may mimic CFIDS symptoms.
3. For at least the past 6 months, I have experienced recurring or persisting:
   a. chills or mild fever; rash over one year that comes and goes
   b. sore throats
   c. painful or swollen lymph glands
   d. unexplained general muscle weakness
   e. fatigue for 24 hours after previously tolerated exercise
   f. headaches unlike any previously experienced
   g. joint pain without joint swelling or redness
   h. forgetfulness
   i. excessive irritability
   j. confusion
   k. inability to concentrate
   l. depression
   m. disturbed sleep

If you answered yes to questions one and two and marked at least eight of the criteria in question 3, then you may have CFIDS.

Criteria developed by The Centers for Disease Control and Prevention.

A PROGRAM TO RESTORE YOUR CHILD'S HEALTH

Wanting to help our little people, Dr. Bland and his team developed a children's medical food product called Ultracare for Kids. Kids can be finicky eaters, so a study was designed including thirty-nine children from the ages of 2 to 11 years to taste the product. Overall 85 percent of the children found the taste acceptable.[4] Currently the mainstream of treatment for food hypersensitivity is the elimination diet. The most common foods to which children react are milk, eggs, peanuts, soy, fish, and wheat. Hypersensitivity reactions to food may contribute to or cause dermatitis (eczema), dysfunctional gastrointestinal disorders, attention deficit hyperactivity disorders, and asthma.[5-8] Elimination of common irritating foods alone may not make the children well, however.

In the tolerance study, children who received the low allergy diet along with the medical food showed significantly more clinical improvement as compared to children who received the diet alone. Overall, 74 percent of the children reported a greater than 20 percent decrease in symptoms. Symptoms such as headaches; itchy or watery eyes; swollen eyelids, tongue, gums, or lips; runny or stuffy nose; joint or muscle aches; rashes; coughing; gastrointestinal complaints; and a variety of other symptoms were evaluated for improvement. In addition, the Symptoms Inventory surveys organ systems and includes energy, mind, and emotion categories for measures of fatigue, hyperactivity, restlessness, and irritability, among other observable changes in behavior. In two case reports, in which the children presented with

attention deficit hyperactivity disorder, improvement in behavior and clinical symptoms were observed after including
Ultracare for Kids. Atopic conditions, such as eczema, were
also improved with this protocol and an elimination diet
program.[9]

CHAPTER 11

CLEANSING THE LIVER AND THE LYMPH SYSTEM

CLEANSING THE LIVER

In addition to the other recommendations I have made for cleansing, a good liver cleanse is of great benefit. Every nutrient and toxin that is absorbed into your blood from your GI tract must pass through the portal vein into the liver before your blood can enter the general circulation. Your liver is the primary site for poison control in your body. Hundreds of different reactions proceed here to keep you safe from dangerous chemicals. It is easiest on your body to do a liver flush after completing a program that addresses your colon health. If you attempt to do a liver cleanse when you have a toxic bowel, you will be dumping toxic contents from your liver into an already toxic environment. Under these circumstances you are virtually guaranteed to get sick from liver detoxification.

If you cleanse your colon first, you cut down on the waste and toxins that your liver has to deal with; your liver gets a break so it has an opportunity to heal better on its own.

Our livers have an amazing capacity to heal. If 80 percent of your liver is destroyed, it will grow back and work for you again. This may have something to do with the abundant amount of blood delivered to this vital organ of detoxification. Your liver gets 20 percent of your blood supply, even though it weighs only about four pounds.

Dietary Changes to Cleanse the Liver

What you put into your mouth is number one. Fried and greasy foods are challenging for your liver to process, especially because of the damaging qualities of most of the commercially available fats and oils. Alcohol is another substance that commands a lot of attention from your liver. Artificial ingredients put a particular stress on your system because they are man-made chemicals. Our bodies have had time to adapt to and benefit from the chemicals in plants and animals with which we have shared the earth for hundreds of thousands of years, but those that just came off of the chemist's shelf present untested and unknown dangers to our health. Eliminating these three classes of foodstuffs and beverage stress will give your liver a break and allow it to begin the process of repair. Also, you would benefit by eliminating or minimizing refined carbohydrates from your diet, such as sugar, white bread, rolls, pasta, pastries, cakes, and cookies.

Eating foods and herbs that are nourishing for your liver is the next step. The green leafy tops of beets are one of the best foods for your liver. You can steam them just like spinach, and put a little lemon on them if you like. They're healthy and delicious. Or you can put the small young leaves in a salad for a new taste sensation and a little added color. A little extra virgin olive oil, especially from a small company that takes special care in pressing their oils, can be helpful for your liver. People who do liver flushes use this oil after a period of fat avoidance to stimulate the gallbladder to contract and flush out gallstones. I no longer recommend the olive oil challenge after a fat avoidance type of liver flush because of the possibility of stressing your system beyond repair.

A colleague decided to do a liver flush on general cleansing principles, even though she had no overt signs of liver stress. Doing that flush, however, started a cascade of events that has caused her to become disabled and to give up her practice. If you decide to go ahead with the olive oil challenge after a fat avoidance type of flush, I would highly recommend first doing a Functional Liver Detoxification Profile with Great Smokies Diagnostic Laboratory to analyze the functional capacity of your liver. If your liver is having a challenge with detoxifying the toxins you are exposed to, you would benefit from a more gentle cleanse and the support of a health-care practitioner. (See appendix 1 for more information.)

Drinking lemon squeezed into water first thing in the morning is a good tonic for your liver. You may also add fresh-squeezed lemon to your water throughout the day for a refreshing alkalizing drink. Stress and the Standard American Diet (SAD) make your body acidic. An alkalizing cordial called Alkaline Broth (page 238) and some of the relaxation techniques such as The Inner Smile recommended in chapter 15 help neutralize acid build up, which leads to dysfunction and disease in your body.

In the case of breaking up gallstones, however, mallic acid from apples is helpful. This acid softens the sludge in your gallbladder so that it flows more easily into your small intestine, then out of your body through elimination. Mallic acid is available in all apple products such as applesauce, unfiltered apple juice, and baked, poached, or raw apples. It is not present in filtered apple juices. Mallic Acid is also available in supplement form, sometimes in conjunction with magnesium, for those who do not like or tolerate apples or apple products.

A combination of equal parts of fennel, anise, and fenugreek seed tea is cleansing to the liver and soothing to your digestive tract. The time you take to brew the tea and drink it can also be a time of quiet reflection and relaxation that will benefit your health.

Nutritional Products for Liver Cleansing

For an added cleansing bonus, you may opt to add nutritional products to your liver cleanse program. There is plenty of research, as was discussed in chapter 9, to show the efficacy of milk thistle, also called Silymarin, in liver support. Milk thistle is plentiful in South America and, surprisingly, on my California hillside. Milk thistle products come in several forms, such as tincture, tablet, and capsule forms in health food stores. All of the products are from the small hard seeds of the plant. If you want to collect some milk thistle seeds for yourself, you need very sturdy gloves, because sharp spines that will penetrate most garden gloves surround seeds. In the case of this herb, it is probably better to purchase a properly prepared and concentrated extract! Milk thistle seed extract standardized to contain 80 percent Silymarin has been proven effective in many years of research. (For suppliers of these products check appendix 1.)

There is also a new form of milk thistle seed extract now available, which offers greater liver protection activity in the body. It is a patented extract standardized to contain 33 percent silybin (the most active part of Silymarin) in a soybean phosphatidylcholine base. It is available from Yerba Prima. See appendix 1 for ordering information.

Some say that taking herbs continuously diminishes their effect. My recommendation is to use the supplement for a period of no more than 2 months straight. If you have serious deterioration of your liver and need to take milk thistle for a prolonged amount of time, you may try taking weekends off, with the consent of your health-care practitioner, to ensure its effectiveness.

A combination vitamin/mineral/amino acid product called Detoxification Factors is helpful in supporting liver detoxification. I have not found it to be as effective as engaging in a thorough cleanse (a modified elimination diet devoid of the usual allergens and with therapeutic food powders), but it is an acceptable compromise for those who cannot or do not wish to engage in a more intensive program. Detoxification Factors (Integrative Therapeutics) include the nutrients needed to support both phases of liver detoxification. It is available through health care practitioners' offices.

Phosfood, a liquid phosphoric acid compound made by Standard Process and available through doctors' offices, helps liquefy the cholesterol-rich sludge that can get trapped in your gallbladder as a result of bad diet and impaired gastrointestinal function. Please use this product only under the supervision of a licensed health care professional.

Because different products have different potencies and concentrations, it is impossible for me to recommend a dosage for the aforementioned products. If you are unsure how to proceed after reading the label directions, ask a knowledgeable clerk or work with the aid a licensed health care professional. The advice I give you is not intended to substitute for medical attention, but intended to be informational only.

Liver Detoxification with Ultra Clear or Ultra Clear Plus

Because some people have sensitivity reactions to herbal products, they are unable to use herbal formulations for cleansing. They would do better with a therapeutic food program using Ultra Clear products. For more information about Ultra Clear products, see chapter 10: "Therapeutic Food Powders for Cleansing."

CLEANSING THE LYMPH SYSTEM

In the early 1900s, an osteopath named Chapman found that by rubbing certain spots on his patients' bodies, he could relieve their pain and improve the health of their organs. These spots became known as Chapman's or Neurolymphatic Reflexes. (For more information, see appendix 1.)

Exercising the Lymph System

One of the best exercises for stimulating lymphatic flow is bouncing on a mini-trampoline jogger. The heel of your foot goes lower than the ball of your foot while you are bouncing on the mini-trampoline. Because of this pulling action, it is perhaps the most effective type of exercise for your lymph system and to stimulate circulation in general. Your lymph does not have a pump like your blood vessels have with your heart. The only direct way to get the lymph system to increase its flow, other than skin brushing (see chapter 15) and massage, is to exercise. When the big muscles of your body contract with exercise, it squeezes your lymph vessels and improves fluid flow.

Of course any form of exercise or movement beyond sitting on the couch and surfing channels with the remote is helpful for encouraging lymph circulation. When you move in any manner, muscles in your body contract and release, squeezing the blood and lymph vessels inside.

CHAPTER 12

MAINTAINING HEALTHIER BOWELS

BOWEL MOVEMENT PROGRESS CHART

Following is a chart that will help you monitor the results of your own cleansing program. I suggest you begin your diary a few days before beginning your cleansing program. This will help you see the dramatic difference that cleansing makes in your daily elimination. If you wish to continue your diary beyond four weeks, just make a photocopy of the page. This is your personal diary, and it will be a valuable motivational tool to keep you inspired to cleanse. Things to watch for and to note on your chart are:

- unusual colors of stool
- amount and bulkiness of stool
- sticky vs. dry stool
- firm vs. loose stool
- floating vs. non-floating stool
- mucus strands or pockets
- other items expelled with stool

DAY	1st Bowel Movement	2nd Bowel Movement	3rd Bowel Movement	4th Bowel Movement	5th Bowel Movement
SUNDAY	TIME: DESCRIPTION:	TIME: DESCRIPTION:	TIME: DESCRIPTION:	TIME: DESCRIPTION:	TIME: DESCRIPTION:
MONDAY	TIME: DESCRIPTION:	TIME: DESCRIPTION:	TIME: DESCRIPTION:	TIME: DESCRIPTION:	TIME: DESCRIPTION:
TUESDAY	TIME: DESCRIPTION:	TIME: DESCRIPTION:	TIME: DESCRIPTION:	TIME: DESCRIPTION:	TIME: DESCRIPTION:
WEDNESDAY	TIME: DESCRIPTION:	TIME: DESCRIPTION:	TIME: DESCRIPTION:	TIME: DESCRIPTION:	TIME: DESCRIPTION:
THURSDAY	TIME: DESCRIPTION:	TIME: DESCRIPTION:	TIME: DESCRIPTION:	TIME: DESCRIPTION:	TIME: DESCRIPTION:
FRIDAY	TIME: DESCRIPTION:	TIME: DESCRIPTION:	TIME: DESCRIPTION:	TIME: DESCRIPTION:	TIME: DESCRIPTION:
SATURDAY	TIME: DESCRIPTION:	TIME: DESCRIPTION:	TIME: DESCRIPTION:	TIME: DESCRIPTION:	TIME: DESCRIPTION:

Figure 12.1 Weekly Bowel Movement Record

Constipation and Laxatives

Forty million Americans currently use laxatives, and 8 million use them at least once a week. Most of these are stimulant laxatives that work by irritating the walls of the intestinal tract, causing increased movement of the colon walls as the body attempts to expel the laxative. With continued use, this results in poor muscle tone, faulty peristalsis, and a further dependence on laxatives. In fact, many people who overuse laxatives reach the point where they are incapable of having a bowel movement without resorting to the use of laxatives, enemas, or colonics. Laxative overuse can also lead to depletion of potassium and other nutrients in the body, as well as to kidney damage in extreme cases.

When constipation does occur, I recommend use of a high-fiber supplement to provide bulk and moisture for smooth elimination rather than turning to stimulant laxatives (see chapters 3 and 7 for more information on dietary fiber). Wheat bran has become popular for achieving regularity, but with repeated use it tends to be harsh and even irritating to the intestinal tact. Also the phytate in wheat bran forms strong bonds with iron and other minerals, thereby reducing their absorption into the body. Psyllium husks are one of the best types of fiber available. They act gently as they form soft, bulky stools, and they are more efficient at removing waste and toxins from the digestive system than other forms of fiber. In rare cases, it may become necessary to consult with a physician. if working with these recommendations and an alternative health-care practitioner has not yielded the results you need.

Sometimes peristalsis just won't work; either it does not occur or is ineffective. If this is the case, drug intervention may be necessary. Waning hormones may also be responsible for a sluggish bowel, as I have mentioned earlier. To support the hormone estrogen's activity, you can add soy products to your diet on a daily basis in the form of tofu, soy milk, soy burgers (one of my staples while finishing the manuscript for this book), soy nuts, tempeh, miso, and so on. Insufficient thyroid hormone activity may also be responsible for a sluggish intestinal tract. Many natural therapies are now available that can increase the secretion of your own hormones and protect the ones that are being produced. A Health Coach, chiropractor, acupuncturist, naturopath, or certified clinical nutritionist may be able to help you in this area. A few medical doctors are also learning about these less invasive and less harmful ways to support hormone balance, although some will freely admit that their patients know more in this area than they do.

It is in your best interest to prevent problems from occurring by maintaining a high-fiber diet and healthy intestinal flora, and by performing a thorough internal cleansing periodically to remove old encrusted waste and improve the health of your elimination system and your entire body. (See chapter 7 for more on high-fiber diet and healthy intestinal flora.)

A NOTE ON COLONICS

A colonic is an enema done with water under pressure, which allows the water to penetrate farther into the large intestine. The colonic is administered by a technician who regulates the water pressure. During an internal cleansing program, an occasional enema or a series of colonics can be helpful in removing impacted waste from the colon, relieving constipation, and assisting the cleansing process. Colonic therapists have found that colonics by themselves are not completely effective in removing the long-term putrefactive matter that has adhered to the intestinal walls for years. However, in conjunction with an herbal cleansing, colonics shorten the time required to remove loosened, impacted matter from the colon wall. Many colonic therapists recommend an herbal cleansing to their patients and are amazed at the amount and content of toxic material released by combining internal cleansing with colonics.

It is easy to disrupt the valuable population of bifidobacteria (bifs) and lactobacteria and to introduce a foreign species that may even lead to death when doing colonics, so precautions must be taken. Make sure the colon therapist uses tubes that are new—and reserved only for you if you return for repeat colonics. Always use properly filtered or distilled water rather than spring or chlorinated water. Spring water may contain unknown microorganisms that could damage your health. When you take water in through your mouth, your digestive juices have the chance to kill off any potential pathogens. But with a colonic, the water is going up the back end of your digestive tract, so you don't have that digestive advantage. And chlorinated water kills off the good bacteria in your intestines. After all, isn't that the job of chlorine in our drinking water—to kill microorganisms? If your therapist does not follow your internal washing with an "implant" of beneficial bacteria, follow the enema or colonic with some of the probiotic supplements mentioned in chapter 14. These may be taken orally.

"GOOD" BACTERIA

Lactobacilli and bifidobacteria (bifs) are our friends. They play a significant role in controlling the pH of the large intestine through the liberation of lactic acid and acetic acid, which in turn restrict the growth of potential pathogens in your gut. Their supportive properties may include production of organic acids that inhibit the growth of certain undesirable bacteria, promotion of normal gastrointestinal function, and promotion of a healthy intestinal wall, to name a few. Bifs are believed to have cancer-protective and cholesterol-lowering properties, as well as the ability to synthesize B-vitamins and vitamin K. All beneficial bacteria are susceptible to eradication, especially through the use of any antibiotics. Sugar in your diet in the form of sweeteners and alcohol supports the overgrowth of yeast such as *Candida,* which damages your intestinal wall and leads to allergies and toxicity. These yeasts can mimic your own cells so that your immune system begins to attack your thyroid gland, heart, or other vital body parts. This simple habit of eating too much sugar or having too many alcoholic drinks can lead to autoimmune disease.

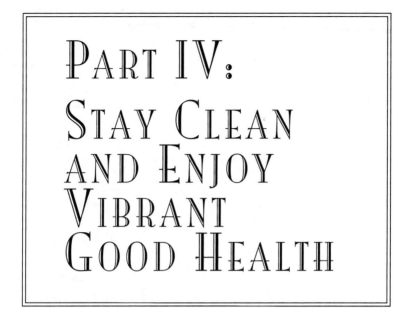

PART IV:

STAY CLEAN AND ENJOY VIBRANT GOOD HEALTH

CHAPTER 13

DIET AND RECIPES THAT COMPLEMENT CLEANSING

"The goal in life is to die young—as late as possible."   — *Ashley Montague, Ph.D.*

WHAT TO EAT?

Using food to heal is not new to health care. The oldest documented medical practice from ancient India, Ayurveda, recognizes three main body types or *doshas*, each responding best, with regards to health, to different foods and lifestyles. For thousands of years, the Chinese have utilized the Five Element Theory, based on the forces of yin and yang with appropriate foods and herbs for each season to create balanced health. Nutritional therapy in Europe is at least two thousand years old. In 400 B.C., Hippocrates wrote about attempts to treat night blindness by increasing the intake of liver. (Today we can pinpoint the substance in liver that helps prevent night blindness: vitamin A.)[1]

As we get farther away from our ancient health-care traditions, the cost of health care is skyrocketing. National health-care expenditures for 1990 alone totaled $666 billion, of which 30 percent has been attributed to conditions associated with inadequate diet. Dietary factors are associated with five of the 10 leading causes of death including coronary heart disease, certain types of cancer, stroke, non-insulin-dependent diabetes mellitus, and atherosclerosis.[2] The major cancers associated with dietary habits are those of the postmenopausal breast, distal colon, prostate, pancreas, ovary, and endometrium. Current evidence suggests that the genotoxic carcinogens for all but the last two of these diseases stem from the intake of fried and broiled foods such as meats. Fish-eating populations have lower incidences of heart disease and of many forms of cancers than do other populations, which may result from the omega-3 oils found in fish. Among other dietary practices that may reduce the risk of cancer and cardiovascular disease are consuming five to nine servings per day of fruits and vegetables (which provide nutrient-dense, high-fiber food) and drinking 2.5 liters of fluids daily. The American Dietetic Association's opinion is that the public must heed this information to achieve long-term health.[3] Researchers have found that phytochemicals and food components have been linked with the prevention and/or treatment of cancer, diabetes, cardiovascular disease, hypertension, osteoporosis, abnormal bowel function, and arthritis as well as many other chronic conditions.[4] A 1996 article from *Nutrition Reviews* reports that the risk of colon and rectal cancer is increased by the intake of saturated fat or animal fat and that the intake of fiber and vegetable products decrease risk.[5]

Bal and Foerster report, "Two-thirds of cancer cases are associated with two lifestyle practices: 35 percent with the typical American diet, and 30 percent with tobacco use." In the results section of their article, they state that there is scientific agreement that dietary goals for the year 2000 include increasing fruit and vegetable consumption to five or more servings per day, increase both cereals and legumes to six or more servings per day, and decrease fat to no more that 30 percent of total calories. However, the authors are pessimistic about Americans making the necessary dietary and lifestyle changes to decrease suffering and death from cancer.[6] Prove them wrong!

In a study at the Ohio State University College of Medicine, 292 of 322 infants less than one year of age, all diagnosed with respiratory allergy, were found to have significant reduction of symptoms following six weeks placement on a hypoallergenic formula containing no milk, egg, wheat, or food additives.[7] Perhaps if we begin to educate and feed our children better, there will be a chance for change. Read further for the results of the High 5 Project, which succeeded in increasing the fruit and vegetable consumption of fourth graders.

Because we all have different food preferences, I do not recommend one nutritional plan for everyone. Rather, I have compiled a list of 10 recommendations that you may incorporate into your daily diet. These suggestions will help you develop a meal plan as a basis for keeping your intestinal tract clean. (If you wish, you may follow the suggested menus on pages 244–247.)

1. Drink plenty of plain, pure water every day. If you do not yet have a source of purified water, in most circumstances it is better to drink tap water than not to drink water at all.
2. Eat plenty of fresh vegetables. They are easy to digest and they provide essential nutrients and fiber. Vegetable juices are excellent for cleansing

your body. Choosing organically grown vegetables
is, of course, your best course of action.

3. Eat plenty of fresh fruit. Fruit is high in vitamins
   and easy to digest, and it helps cleanse your body.
   Keep intake of fruit to a minimum if you are hypoglycemic or carbohydrate intolerant (see Determining Your Sensitivity to Insulinogenic Foods and
   Eating Habits, chapter 8) — especially sweet fruits
   such as bananas, sweet melon, dates, and grapes.
   Again, organically grown fruit is your best choice.

4. Eat whole grains if you tolerate them. People with
   A and AB blood types have the least trouble. Whole
   grains (as opposed to refined grains) are high in
   dietary fiber and contain an acceptable balance of
   proteins, carbohydrates, vitamins, minerals, and
   natural oils. Try adding some grains that are new
   to a North American's diet. Quinoa and amaranth
   are ancient grains from South America. They are
   higher in protein than our standard wheat, corn,
   and rice, and because you were probably not exposed to them in your tender youth, they are unlikely to cause sensitivities or allergies in your
   system. In the following pages, I have included
   recipes that incorporate both of these nourishing
   grains.

5. Eat more sprouted grains, beans, and seeds. They
   are excellent sources of enzymes, protein, and fiber,
   and as an added bonus, they are packed with vitamins and minerals. Because they are "alive," your
   body has an easier time digesting and assimilating
   sprouted foods. If you have a weak digestive system, you may not be able to tolerate raw food. If

that is the case, steam your sprouts, vegetables, and fruits to a tenderness suitable to the current health of your digestive tract.

6. Eat plenty of beans and soy products. They are high in protein and fiber and are excellent complements to grains. To reduce the gas-forming properties of beans, you can use a product called Bean-O. It contains the enzyme raphinose, which breaks down the indigestible fiber portion of beans that causes gas. The macrobiotic community also claims that cooking a couple of sheets of kombu seaweed at the bottom of your pot of beans helps to eliminate gas. Be sure to soak the dry beans, then throw out the soaking water and rinse the beans to assist this process. Because I don't eat many dairy products, and I rarely have an egg, I have invented some whipped cream substitutes and pudding recipes using tofu (which is made from soybeans) to satisfy those desires for creamy, sweet food (see recipes on pages 239–241).

7. Eat raw, organically grown nuts and seeds. They are high in protein, oils, and valuable minerals. They are best eaten in moderation—no more than a handful at any one time—because they are so concentrated. Whole nuts that still contain their germ lend themselves to sprouting. Sunflower seeds with the shells on can be grown like a grass; they make a delicious, nutty sprout treat (often available in supermarkets or health food stores). Raw almonds, hazelnuts, and sunflower seeds without the shell are more digestible if soaked overnight in pure water. Organically grown nuts

are much healthier than nuts grown with pesticides, and they should be stored in your freezer or refrigerator in a tightly sealed container to protect their abundant oils from becoming rancid. If you have herpes, you may want to strictly limit your intake of nuts and seeds. (*Note:* Nuts, seeds, and grains, especially corn, are high in arginine, which feeds the herpes virus. You can counteract the arginine with lysine or eating concentrated dairy products like yogurt or cottage cheese.)

8. Eat plenty of cultured or fermented dairy products such as yogurt, kefir, and buttermilk if you tolerate them. If you are unsure, buy a small container as a trial. They are easier to digest than milk, and they usually contain lactobacteria that are beneficial to your intestinal tract. Remember to get organic or non-fat versions that say "live cultures" on the label for your best health. I also recommend that you look for statements on the container that say something like, "The milk used to make this product came from cows that were not treated with bovine somatotropic hormone (BSH)." Unless you want to grow up to be like a cow, you don't need extra cow hormones in your diet.

9. Eat fish. It's a good source of protein and essential fatty acids (EFAs). Because our planet is increasingly polluted, there are concerns (especially for pregnant women) about the toxins that are concentrated in fish. We discussed at length the dangers of eating any fish from the Great Lakes. However, ocean fish generally have a high concentration of selenium, which binds the toxins and makes them

harmless to your body when you eat them. You can also buy farm-raised fish, which may be a cleaner product, but the fish may be laden with antibiotic residue utilized in the fish farming process. Call your fish market and ask what the farm-raised fish are fed. If they are fed fish pellets made from mackerel, cod, herring, or other fish, then your fish should be fine. If they are fed grains or chicken parts, don't buy them. If you do regular cleansing, eat a diet high in EFAs, fruit, and vegetables, drink pure water, and think good thoughts, the benefits of eating fish two to four times per week will probably outweigh the dangers you may encounter. Choose the high-EFA fish that I recommended in chapter 3.

10. Take a fiber supplement from psyllium, flax, barley, oat, rice, or a combination; a probiotic formula; and omega-3 EFAs such as flaxseed oil or EPA/DHA daily for a well-balanced nutritional program. It is unlikely that food will give you all of the nutrition you need for optimum health even if you are mindful of your diet. The benefits of these supplements have been discussed in detail in chapters 7 and 9.

Phytonutrients

Phyto comes from a Greek word meaning "plant." Phytonutrients are plant-derived substances that are highly active in the body. More than 20,000 such nutrients in plants have been identified; they not only give plants their bright colors but also protect the plants and those of us who eat them from environmental stressors. Plant foods typically contain 25 to 200 percent more minerals than animal foods.[8] One-third of all enzymes in the body require minerals to do their work. A diet rich in fresh fruits, vegetables, nuts, seeds, grains, and legumes contains hundreds of special compounds that promote good health and are associated with a lowered risk of heart disease, diabetes, high blood pressure, obesity, and cancer. Two recent articles support the use of potassium, magnesium, and fruits and vegetables to increase bone density, which makes bones stronger and less likely to fracture as we age.[9,10] Phytonutrients help reduce our risk of developing these conditions and diseases through antioxidant activity, hormone regulation, suppression of inflammatory pathways, and support of detoxification pathways that flush out carcinogens.

In a 1992 article titled "The Role of Dietary Phytosterols in Colon Carcinogenesis" that appeared in *Nutrition and Cancer*, researchers headed by A. V. Rao stated, "For most cancer sites, persons with low fruit and vegetable intake (at least the lower one-fourth of the population) experience about twice the risk of cancer compared with those with high intake, even after control for potentially confounding factors."[11] A study being undertaken by Britain's Imperial Cancer Research Fund and the Medical Research Council finds, after 17 years, that people who eat fresh fruit daily are 24 percent less likely to die from a heart attack; strokes decrease by 32 percent, and 21 percent are less likely to die in any given year. This study was confirmed by the Framingham Heart Study, which found that eating three additional servings daily of fruits and vegetables reduced overall stroke rates 22 percent and the risk of bleeding stroke by 51 percent.[12]

In a recent study at the University of Alabama, fourth graders in 28 elementary schools were fed an increased amount of fruits and vegetables. Reynolds, and the team of researchers stated that, "Strong effects were found for the High 5 intervention on fruit and vegetable consumption, on macro- and micronutrients, and on psychosocial variables."[13] Which means that when the children ate more produce, they were better nourished and better behaved. Would that be a benefit in your household?

In addition to their individual healing properties, most phytonutrients are antioxidants that trap pollution particles known as free radicals. They have also been shown to stop cancer-causing enzymes from performing their dastardly work.

HEALING FOODS FROM NATURE'S BOUNTY

Eat rainbow colored foods. What colors show up on your table? Here are some examples of foods' healing properties.

Red grapes, blackberries, blueberries, and cherries get their royal colors from *anthocyanins,* powerful antioxidants that dilate blood vessels, aid vision, and may help prevent heart disease and stroke. According to a recent Tufts study, eating blueberries dramatically reversed memory loss and restored motor coordination and balance in aged animals. You would eat about half a cup a day to equal the animals' dosage, or you can take a standardized extract of bilberry (blueberry) fruit, 160 to 320 milligrams per day. Yerba Prima makes a 160-milligram capsule of bilberry using the same extract used in the medical studies.

Blackberries, blueberries, raspberries, and strawberries possess a trio of nutrients—phenolic acids, catechins, and flavonoids—that trap free radicals, stop harmful enzymes, and normalize hormones. Flavonoids also protect your eyes and your heart.

Kiwi fruit has three hundred times as much vitamin C as a comparable weight of oranges, and it is loaded with potassium and the good enzymes bromelain and papain, which help injured tissue to heal. Kiwis are also effective for removing excess sodium from the body, which is helpful for people with sodium-dependent high blood pressure.

Mint contains powerful phytonutrients (plant nutrients) called monoterpenes, antioxidants that stimulate protective enzyme production. It is easy to grow mint in a pot or in your yard for a fresh supply whenever you want it. Citrus peel and caraway seeds are other monoterpene food sources.

Peaches and melons grace us with beta-carotene, which is also present in other yellow and orange fruits and vegetables, as well as in leafy greens. Researchers think that beta-carotene is a marker for a wide range of other phytonutrients. There are 600 known carotenoid antioxidants. Honeydew melons have blood-thinning properties to protect your cardiovascular system.

Citrus fruits feed you folic acid in addition to their well-known vitamin C content. They also contain liminoids and terpenes, which stimulate protective enzymes, including ones that block carcinogenic activities in your body. Later in this chapter, look for some delicious recipes high in these colorful and nutrition-packed foods.

Broccoli, cauliflower, cabbage, and brussels sprouts are cruciferous vegetables that contain the phytonutrients indole and sulfurophane. Indoles may support healthy estrogen metabolism in your body, thereby helping to protect women against breast and ovarian cancers. Sulfurophanes support the removal of toxins and carcinogens, protecting DNA from damage. Glusinolates, the parent compound of sulfurophanes, have the ability to improve the detoxification ability of the liver and other organs to render chemicals, drugs, and pollutants harmless.[14,15]

Soybeans contain phytoestrogens that may help to normalize your body's hormonal balance. In this way, they may protect against hormone-related cancers such as breast and prostate cancer. In countries where a lot of soybean foods are consumed, the incidence of hormone-related cancers is low.

Garlic, onions, leeks, and chives contain allyl sulfides that support cardiovascular health and optimal cholesterol levels. Some studies link these foods to a lower incidence of stomach and colon cancer as well.

Green tea is rich in polyphenols—bioflavonoids with powerful antioxidant properties. It is a favorite beverage of the Japanese, who have a low incidence of gastric cancers.

Tomatoes, red grapefruit, watermelon, and apricots are full of lycopenes—antioxidants with twice the activity of beta-carotene. A study reported in the *International Journal of Cancer* showed that the group of people who ate the most tomatoes had half the risk of digestive tract cancers (mouth, throat, esophagus, stomach, colon, and rectal) of the group who ate the least. Another study found that men who ate at least 10 servings of tomato-based foods per week reduced their risk of developing prostate cancer by 45 percent.

Carrots, corn, pumpkin, and squash are high in beta-carotene. Diets rich in this nutrient have been linked to a reduced risk of heart disease and cancer. Beta-carotene promotes the production of vitamin A, which supports your immune system.

Spinach, collard greens, kale, and parsley are rich in another class of carotenoids: lutein and zeaxanthin. These are pigments found in the macula of your eyes. The macula is in the central part of the retina and contains the greatest concentration of nerve cells so that you can see. Macular degeneration is a major cause of blindness in the elderly. If you have this condition, you lose the central part of your vision and can see only in the periphery or outside edges of your field of vision. An article published in the *Journal of the American Medical Association* showed a relationship between macular degeneration and diets low in lutein and zeaxanthin.

Herbs have a variety of phytonutrients that have been used to restore health throughout the ages. Some more widely recognized herbs are ginger root, milk thistle seed, turmeric, echinacea, dong quai, and ginkgo. These herbs have traditionally been used as antispasmodics or to support the liver and the digestive and immune systems. Some herbs are known for their use as adaptogens—nutrients that help us adapt to the physical and mental stressors of a modern lifestyle.

Astragalus root, aloe vera, and many Chinese mushrooms contain polysaccharides, which support immune system function.

Horseradish, mustard, cabbage, turnips, and cashew nuts contain isothiocyanates, which support detoxification and the removal of carcinogens.

Lentils and beans are rich in saponins, which help reduce the growth of cancer cells.

Spirulina, chlorella, and dunaliella are "superfoods" in a class called microalgae. They contain a wide range of the amino acids, carbohydrates, EFAs, vitamins, and minerals we need to support life. They are the richest known vegetarian source of vitamin B_{12}. Microalgae are the lowest food on the food chain, making life out of only sunlight, water, and the minerals floating in the aquatic environment in which they grow. The addition of Earthrise Spirulina to my diet was one of the most significant steps I have ever taken toward improving my health.

Flower pollen is another superfood that provides protein, carbohydrates, EFAs, enzymes, coenzymes, vitamins, and minerals. It also contains flavonoids, polyphenols, carotenoids, and other phytonutrients. Many people who eat this superfood report improved energy levels.

CLEANSING DIET

The 20-Day Rejuvenation Diet Program contains what is described as a diet plan designed to improve the health and vitality of the average individual who feels he or she is aging too fast, does not have the level of energy he or she would like, or is plagued by everyday minor aches and pains. Dr. Jeffrey Bland and colleagues conducted a study with twenty-four individuals using the 20-day diet protocol. Between 81 and 100 percent reported "overall satisfaction" during the final 13 days of the diet. A significant decrease in Medical Symptoms Questionnaire (MSQ) scores was observed after the diet program. In addition, an increase in quality of life parameters was also noted, as assessed by the Medical Outcomes Survey (MOS) SF-36 Health Status Survey. In general, individuals found the diet experience to be satisfactory, the menus to provide tasty meals, and the program to improve energy and general health. In addition to the diet, subjects were asked to consume an over-the-counter multivitamin and antioxidant supplement daily.

The authors of *The 20-Day Rejuvenation Diet Program* (see appendix 1) suggest that individuals who will obtain the most benefit from the diet are those who report MSQ scores between 25 and 100. They suggest that individuals scoring above 100 should visit a practitioner, whereas individuals who score below 25 are considered to have modest health concerns and may not observe a change in symptoms.[16]

ALOE VERA

The aloe vera plant is a succulent and a member of the lily family. Aloe vera leaves are filled with a healthful inner gel that contains many valuable nutrients, including vitamins, minerals, enzymes, lipids (fats), amino acids, and healing mucopolysaccharides. Aloe vera has been known for centuries as an overall curative and an almost "miracle working" plant. Dioscorides, a medical practitioner in the first century, made a detailed report on aloe for treating wounds, insomnia, stomach disorders, general pain, constipation, and many other disorders. But Western civilization lost the knowledge of aloe as a healing substance until recently.

During the past 50 years, much research on aloe vera has been undertaken to determine why it was so valued throughout history. The studies reveal that aloe vera is very effective in supporting the process of healing from many ailments, including burns, gum disease, and hemorrhoids. One of the greatest benefits of aloe vera juice is the soothing and cleansing effect it has on the whole digestive system. It relieves inflammation of the stomach, especially in the case of ulcers. Research has also shown that aloe inhibits the growth of both staphylococcus and coliform bacteria—the "bad guys"—and promotes the growth of the good lactobacteria that are essential for good digestion.

Aloe vera is particularly beneficial when following an internal cleansing program. At the beginning and for several weeks after ending a program, take 2 to 4 ounces of aloe vera juice per day. The cleansing process can be stimulating and irritating for some people. Properly prepared aloe juice helps to soothe the stomach and entire digestive system with its gentle anti-inflammatory, pain-reducing, and cell-renewing properties. I recommend Quantum Aloe Drink from Premier Research Labs.

CUSTOM NUTRIENT SUPPLEMENTATION

Our body needs nourishment. The need for nourishment is non-negotiable. Our best option is to eat organic foods whenever possible and to take a custom nutritional supplement. Some say, "But I eat a good diet. Why do I need to take supplements?" Consider this: Changes in food growing, harvesting, production, and transportation have resulted in substantial decreases in the vitamin and mineral content of our food supply. Chemical fertilizers and forced growth techniques deplete multiple nutrients from the soil. Fruit is harvested early, then shipped long distances and stored in warehouses for who knows how long before the produce actually reaches your table. The result is that minerals such as calcium, zinc, selenium, and copper are far lower in our foods today as compared to the past. Between 1914 and 1992 the amount of calcium in an apple reduced by 50%, magnesium by 70%, and iron by 90%. Lettuce has 50% less calcium since 1968 and almost no selenium anymore.

Farmed fish are probably deficient in essential fatty acids (EFA's), plus antibiotics are used in their pools to prevent disease from overcrowded conditions. When you eat the fish you're also getting the antibiotics. Depending on getting EFA's from wild fish is tricky since both heavy metals and pesticide residues are present in these. Cows and chickens eat feed that's been sprayed with herbicides and pesticides and grown on depleted soils. Pasteurizing milk decreases its vitamin B12 and B6 content, and if the cow is given growth hormone (all are unless otherwise stated on the label) levels of vitamins A and B decline while synthetic hormone levels rise.

Supplementing with a good multivitamin mineral would seem a logical choice, but that can be difficult. Most commercial preparations are based on meeting the RDI (Reference Daily Intake). The RDI is what's necessary to prevent deficiency diseases but unfortunately not enough to optimize our health and performance. It doesn't take into account common lifestyle habits like dieting, alcohol intake, sleep deficiency, drug/nutrient depletions, and smoking. Nor does it consider individual genetics, pregnancy, PMS, menopause, athletics, or stress. I want more for myself and my family. Don't you?

So what is the solution? My choice and the choice for my family as well as my patients is a web-based, custom nutrition program that utilizes 5,000+ rules from science to adjust what is included and excluded from your personalized nutritional packets and to determine each nutrient's optimal dose. These rules are updated weekly. The program has been developed by the Health Coach team under the brand name NutriScan.

NutriScan's supplements are tailored to each person's unique needs and automatically take into account:

Age	Drug/Nutrient depletions
Gender	Lifestyle habits
Geography	Genetic predispositions
Dietary habits	Circadian rhythms
Current health	Drug/Nutrient interactions
Allergies	Drug/Herb interactions

Health Coach's comprehensive online health assessment was developed by a team of Harvard PhD's, physicians, medical advisers, nutritionists, and dieticians. Your health professional can use this assessment to comprehensively assess your specific biochemical needs. The result is your very own daily Custom Nutrient Packets, containing the precise blend of vitamins, minerals, phytonutrients (plant based nutrients), and enzymes your body requires to support vibrant health. Your NutriScan Custom Packet will replace a multitude of different bottles of supplements, markedly improving convenience and cost effectiveness. NutriScan's proprietary formulas cannot be found anywhere else in the marketplace. Science tells us that those who take supplements for at least ten years are those who benefit the most in terms of good health. Recent studies have also shown properly personalized supplementation outperforms standard multivitamin and mineral approaches.

Doesn't it make sense to engage in a system that is constantly adjusting for the latest in science, is tailored for your safety with respect to nutrient dosages and any contraindications, and comes from the best manufacturers?

Your personalized supplements are shipped directly to your home with your name on each packet indicating the best time of day to take them. NutriScan is the safest, most convenient, and highest quality system I've encountered in my thirty-six-year quest for superior nutrition. (See appendix 1 for more information.)

BENTONITE

Bentonite is a natural clay mineral that exists as discrete deposits in most continents of the world. It was created primarily in volcanic eruptions millions of years ago, when the volcanic ash settled in shallow seas and eventually became bentonite clay. Some of the largest deposits are found in the Great Plains area of the United States.

There are two major types of bentonite, identified by the major exchangeable ion present in the clay. Those higher in sodium, as opposed to calcium, have greater beneficial activity. In its purified form, bentonite is free of all contamination. It passes through your body undigested. This clay is composed of numerous microscopic platelets, each with negative charges on the flat surfaces and positive charges on the edges. When properly hydrated, the water molecules cause these platelets to separate into a porous structure containing both negative and positive charges. This swelling allows bentonite to absorb substances in the space between the platelets. The ionic charges give bentonite the ability to bind toxins and hold them until they are eliminated. The structure of Great Plains Bentonite creates an enormous surface — more than 900 square yards per tablespoon — that traps and binds pesticides and other potentially harmful substances so that they do not remain in your body.

Montmorillonite, the principal constituent of bentonite, is used in many industries, including water treatment, cosmetics, pharmaceuticals, and dietary supplements. Tested against other clays, including kaolin, which is found in Kaopectate, low concentrations of montmorillonite were more effective than high concentrations of other clays in suppressing the activity of a highly infectious fungus called *Histoplasma capsulatum* that is present in soil and can cause lung diseases and other complications when inhaled.

I am happy to announce that bentonite has been found effective in neutralizing pesticides. It is comforting to know that there is a natural antidote to these dangerous synthetic poisons. Bentonite was an effective part of treatment for Paraquat (a pesticide) toxicity, and the toxicity of Roundup (an herbicide) was reduced when bentonite was used. In the mid-1970s, the Committee of Scientists of the Agricultural Research Service, U.S. Department of Agriculture (USDA), listed 169 agricultural pesticides used in the United States. Nearly two-thirds were shown to be potentially adsorbed onto bentonite, neutralizing their toxicity to humans.

Aflatoxins are extremely carcinogenic molds found on grains and nuts, especially peanuts. Although many countries test their grain and peanut products for aflatoxin content, we may still be exposed to tiny amounts of this toxic compound in our diets. Bentonite clay is able to bind with aflatoxin in the digestive system and remove this poison from your body. This is an area where veterinary research is ahead of human research. People who grow and care for cattle, pigs, sheep, and chickens are very concerned about the health of their animals. They have found that aflatoxin harms the proper growth and development of young animals. As a result of years of research with bentonite, growing animals are often fed a small amount of bentonite as part of their daily diet to counteract any potential harm from aflatoxin in their grain feed and to ensure normal growth. Bentonite with a high ratio of sodium ions has been found most effective for removing this toxin.

Bentonite has also been evaluated for its ability to relieve diarrhea. In the 1960s, a liquid solution of bentonite was tested in thirty-five cases of diarrhea caused by virus infection, food allergy, spastic colon, mucous colitis, or food poisoning. The diarrhea cleared up in thirty-four of the thirty-five cases in an average of 4 days by taking 2 tablespoons three times per day. In animal studies in the 1980s, bentonite blocked intestinal absorption of a toxic substance introduced into the food of rats. This toxin is known to cause vomiting, refusal to eat, and gastrointestinal lesions in livestock, poultry, and humans. In another study published in *Gastroenterology*, bentonite was shown to bind to toxins in the blood from *E. coli* and other sources: "The most effective material in the prevention of endotoxemia proved to be bentonite."

In considering which brand of bentonite to choose to augment your cleansing needs, please consider three factors: ion ratios, activity, and purity. Choose a product that has a high ratio of sodium to calcium ions. Maximum swelling and binding activity are achieved when the sodium ions make up 65 to 75 percent of the total exchangeable ions. Use only the highest grade, which is purified USP/NF (United States Pharmacopoeia/National Formulary).

My bentonite of choice is Great Plains Bentonite. It meets or exceeds all of the above criteria. Its purification process goes through many stages. First, water washing removes any non-clay material and then removes the less effective non-swelling fraction of the clay. Finally, the material is dried, milled, sorted, and tested extensively to ensure that it exceeds the stringent USP/NF purity standards for microbial limits, absence of pathogens, absence of adulteration, and product consistency. Every batch of Great Plains Bentonite is tested for purity and consistency.

I have used other forms of bentonite in the past, and I was impressed by the whiteness of the Great Plains product. Does that mean that the product I used before contained impurities? Probably so. The use of advanced processing methods give Great Plains Bentonite a surface area of more than 960 square yards per serving. That is more than 12 football fields of surface area per quart bottle! (See appendix 1 for purchasing information.)

The Importance of Water— *Plenty* of Water

I discussed the value of pure water extensively in chapters 3 and 6. If you are not drinking enough water during a cleanse, you will endanger the health of your tissues as concentrated toxins are being eliminated from your cells. Furthermore, dehydration can have deleterious effects on your body, eventually leading to death. Probably few of us are close to that stage of water loss, but if you are experiencing heartburn, rheumatoid pain, back pain, heart or angina pain, headaches, or leg pain from walking, you may be suffering from chronic dehydration.

Joint movement is facilitated by water. The cartilage lining in your joints needs fluid to create a cushion between your bones. Without sufficient water, an inflammatory process can ensue to compensate for the lack of water. It may appear that there is an infection or arthritis in your joints, when in reality there is only dehydration.

In your stomach and duodenum—the first portion of your small intestine—a mucus barrier prevents acid penetration and damage to your gastrointestinal lining. A well-hydrated mucus barrier will retain bicarbonate and neutralize acid as it tries to pass through the mucus. Hydration will provide a much better acid barrier to the mucosa than any medication on the market.

If your double-layer cell membranes lack sufficient water, enzyme movement into and out of your cells will be obstructed. Enzymes are necessary to activate cell functions.

Even hypertension (high blood pressure) can be helped by optimal water consumption. When you have inadequate volume in your bloodstream, the vessels selectively decrease in diameter. The vascular system adapts to volume loss by selectively closing the blood vessel lumen. One major cause of blood volume loss is insufficient body water. In chronic dehydration, water is lost from inside of some cells, from water volume held outside the cells, and from water held in the blood vessels. The compensatory closing of the lumen to compensate for water loss causes the rise in tension recognized as hypertension.

Drink Half Your Weight in Water Every Day

If you weigh 160 pounds, you would benefit by drinking 80 ounces of water each day. Or if you weigh 200 pounds, then drink 100 ounces of water. The tallest water bottles available at grocery stores contain approximately 52 ounces of water.

If you weigh 104 pounds, that would be the amount of water that would benefit you most. You can also get water in fruit juices, teas, sparkling water, and soda, but each has a distinct disadvantage.

When you drink juice, you are requiring the digestive machinery and the pancreas to fire up and work, whereas pure water allows your body to flush out toxins without mobilizing your digestive system.

Caffeinated tea is actually a diuretic. By drinking caffeinated teas, coffee, colas, and chocolate drinks, you deplete the supply of water available in your body to dilute toxins and "moisturize" your system. Herbal teas often have therapeutic effects that also make your body work instead of giving it a well-deserved rest. Some herbal teas, such as parsley tea, are also diuretic in action.

Sparkling water may have a high level of phosphorus, which can interfere with calcium absorption in your body and contribute to the development of osteoporosis—something we all want to avoid.

Soda is in a class by itself. Read ingredients; they may not be what you want to put in your body. Many sodas are "rich" in toxic synthetic chemicals and caffeine. One can of soda may contain *6 tablespoons* of sugar. In addition, soda may be high in phosphorus and benzene, a carcinogen.

Some people have difficulty drinking water. Here are some suggestions that may help:

- Sip from a small juice glass throughout the day.
- Squeeze fresh lemon juice in your water. It then becomes an alkalinizing treat to help neutralize the acid of many diseases, disorders, or conditions. This

drink will help normalize your pH, enhancing all of
the metabolic processes that your body performs
every second of your life. Patients who formerly
drank a lot of soda told me that they enjoyed this
unsweetened lemonade so much that they didn't
feel deprived from giving up their soda. If you use
Meyer lemons, which are sweeter than normal
lemons, you automatically add to the deliciousness
of this tasty beverage and you gain the benefit of
the naturally occurring vitamin C with your lemon-
charged water.

- Add a slice of cucumber in your water. I was first
  introduced to this refreshing drink in a Mexican
  restaurant. It is also slightly alkalizing.

- Mix a fruit juice that you like with an equal amount
  of water. That way you cause less of a digestive reaction, enjoy a taste sensation that you like, and
  benefit from increased water consumption. You
  may find that, as you become accustomed to this
  new taste, you will be able to increase the proportion of water to juice.

- Soak in a tub of water. Did you ever notice how
  you have to urinate after swimming or soaking in
  water? You absorb water through your skin, which
  is why it is so important to bathe, soak, or shower
  in high-quality water.

Getting good nutrition can be delicious and fun. Following are a few favorite recipes that help me enjoy nutrient-
rich and scrumptious meals. Feel free to improvise. Let your
intuition and available, appealing ingredients be your guides

to preparing delicious, nutritious food for you and your loved ones.

ANTIOXIDANT SALADS

You know by now the importance of having a diet rich in antioxidant nutrients to combat the effects of toxicity from whatever the source: the environment, your own digestive system, or your home or workplace. Eating ripe fruit and vegetables in season is one of the best ways to fulfill this need. If ripe produce is not available, you may purchase frozen fruits and vegetables; these foods are often frozen within hours of picking. Some argue that quick-frozen food is fresher than produce purchased at the supermarket, because supermarket food has been kept in storehouses and shipped across the country or around the world before it finally reaches your table. The best way to be assured of the quality of the food you eat is to grow your own. Because that plan doesn't fit into many busy lifestyles, a local farmers' market is the next best option.

A word about organically grown versus commercially grown produce: Organic is better. Some organically grown foods boast a nutrient density as much as 90 percent higher than commercially grown foods. In order to look pretty and sell quickly, foods require a minimum level of nutrients in the soil in which they grow. This does not ensure that they will have the nutrients necessary to make a human being healthy. Organically grown food usually costs more than commercially grown food, but considering that, on average, it has 50 percent more nutrition than commercial produce, the higher cost is well worth the price. As a bonus, organically grown produce is free of harmful pesticides (see chapter 5 for a discussion of the dangers of pesticides).

Antioxidant Fruit Salad

Yield: 3 to 6 servings

> 2 oranges *or* 1 grapefruit, peeled and sliced
> 2 kiwis, chopped into bite-size pieces
> 2 bananas, chopped into bite-size pieces
> 2 crisp apples, cored and sliced (peeled optional)
> 1 cup blueberries, fresh or frozen*
> 1 fresh pineapple, chopped into bite-size pieces
> 1 cup halved strawberries, fresh or frozen*
> 1 mango, chopped into bite-size pieces

Place the oranges (or grapefruit) and the kiwi in a bowl. Then mix in the other ingredients. The ascorbic acid from the citrus and kiwi will coat the rest of the fruit and protect it from oxidizing (turning brown).

This delicious salad is high in vitamin C, vitamin A, beta-carotene, fiber, *acanthosides* from the blueberries (good for vision), antifungal substances from the banana, and proteolytic enzymes (which can kill parasites and decrease pain and inflammation) from the pineapple, plus whatever other great nutrients we have yet to discover.

Note: If some of the fruit is frozen, microwave it up to 2 minutes or heat over a double boiler until softened; then mix in with the other fruit.

Antioxidant Vegetable Salad

Yield: 2 to 4 servings

    1 to 2 grated or thinly sliced carrots
    ½ onion, thinly sliced or diced, *or* 1 to 2 green onions,
        diced
    1 to 2 stalks celery, thinly sliced
    1 small cucumber, sliced or cubed
    1 red or green pepper, sliced or diced
    1 head broccoli, chopped into florets, raw or slightly
        steamed

Mix all ingredients together. Serve on a bed of raw lettuce
or cooked greens.

This salad is high in vitamin A, vitamin C, beta-
carotene, flavonoids from the onion, and anticarcinogenic
substances from the broccoli, plus whatever else Mother
Nature has provided for us that we don't know about yet!

Lemon and Garlic Salad Dressing

Yield: about 1½ cups

    ½ cup flaxseed oil
    ½ cup sesame oil *or* olive oil
    1 to 2 cloves garlic, crushed or diced
    Juice of 1 lemon *or* 2 limes
    Splash of your favorite vinegar (optional)
    Salt, tamari, soy sauce, or Bragg's Liquid Aminos
        (non-fermented), to taste
    Freshly ground pepper, to taste

Whip together or blend all ingredients, and pour over salad. You may add some mustard or nut butter for a different taste or texture. Sunflower and sesame butter (tahini) are two of my favorites. Avoid peanut butter, because its fat suppresses immune system function.

The EFAs from the oils and seeds are immunity boosting, heart protective, anti-inflammatory, and hormone regulating to enhance your health.

Poppy Seed Dressing

Yield: 6 servings

This recipe and the next two dressings come from Health Coach's Guilt Free Indulgence cookbook. They are all delicious and, with the addition of flaxseed oil, boost your daily supply of health-enhancing EFAs.

Use this dressing for any salad, pita pocket, potato, or pasta salad. Keep the extra dressing in a dark bottle in the refrigerator for future use.

> 2 tablespoons honey
> 2 tablespoons sesame seeds
> 1 tablespoon poppy seeds
> 1½ teaspoons white onion, chopped
> ¼ teaspoon wheat-free tamari/soy sauce *or* Worcestershire sauce
> ¼ teaspoon paprika
> ¼ cup flaxseed oil
> ¼ cup sunflower oil
> ¼ cup cider vinegar (replace with tarragon vinegar or lemon juice for variety)

Simply combine all ingredients in a blender or food processor and process until smooth.

Ginger Dressing

Yield: about ¼ cup

This light dressing is great over grains, lettuce, vegetables, coleslaw, or any other salad. You couldn't ask for anything simpler.

> 3 tablespoons flaxseed oil
> 1 to 2 tablespoons freshly squeezed lemon juice
> 1 teaspoon freshly grated ginger
> 1 clove garlic, minced

Place ingredients in a bowl and whisk together with a fork or blend a larger quantity of all the ingredients in a blender and retain for future use. Store in a dark bottle in the refrigerator.

Lemon-Orange Dressing

Yield: about 2 cups

Extremely easy to make, this is a dressing that can be used for salads, rice, pasta, or any grain dish. With the lemon and orange juice incorporated, it is a dressing filled with sunshine! If you are sensitive to vinegar yet enjoy some zing, then this is perfect for you.

> ¼ cup fresh-squeezed lemon juice
> 3 tablespoons fresh-squeezed orange juice
> ½ cup sunflower oil
> ½ cup flaxseed oil
> 1 tablespoon dill weed *or* 1 teaspoon dried dill
> 1 tablespoon marjoram
> ½ teaspoon fresh ginger root *or* 1 teaspoon ground
>   ginger

Just toss all the ingredients into a blender and mix. Place it in a dark bottle and refrigerate.

HEALTHY GRAINS

These grain recipes are high in omega-3 and omega-6 EFAs.

Instant Hot Cereal

Yield: 2 servings

This simple, fast, yet nutritious cereal from The Guilt Free Gourmet *can be altered quite easily to give you a good variety of flavors. Cool mornings are always a great time for hot cereal, provided you are hungry and looking for something to hold you and yours until noon or at least break time. It is also a favorite afternoon snack.*

> 1½ cups pure water, apple cider, or other fruit juice
> Handful of raisins *and/or* chopped almonds, if desired
> 1 tablespoon sesame seeds *or* sunflower seeds
> ½ cup ground grains such as amaranth, brown rice, oat groats, oat bran, millet, buckwheat groats, or rye (use one or two of these)
> *Toppings* (optional): cinnamon; flaxseed oil; fresh fruit, puréed

Bring the water, cider, or juice to a boil with the raisins, nuts, and seeds, then add the grains, stirring constantly. Simmer for 5 minutes or until desired texture is achieved, and serve. Top it with cinnamon and flaxseed oil or a little fresh fruit purée, such as applesauce. Mmmmm!

Note: It's best to grind your own grains in a coffee or seed grinder, but you can purchase ground grains from your health food store.

Blueberry Oatmeal

Yield: 3 or 4 servings

If you enjoy hot oatmeal on those cold, blizzard-struck mornings, then this will be a real treat for you. It can also be made with other fruits such as strawberries, raspberries, or bananas. This is another recipe from the Guilt Free Indulgence.

2 cups apple cider
1 cup pure water
1 cup rolled oats
3 tablespoons flaxseeds, ground
½ cup rice cereal *or* short-grain rice (ground in your grinder)
Handful of blueberries, raisins, *or* other fruit (fresh or frozen)

Bring the apple cider and water to a boil. Stir in the remaining ingredients and let cook on medium heat for 15 minutes or until done.

Note: Try grinding your own grains in a coffee or seed grinder, or purchase freshly ground grains from your health food store.

Fiber Muffins

Yield: about 2 dozen 2-inch muffins

2 cups whole wheat flour
1 cup Colon Care Formula *or* Nutri Flax
¾ teaspoon unrefined sea salt
1¼ teaspoons baking soda
2 cups plain yogurt, non-fat organic

1 egg, lightly beaten, *or* 2 tablespoons ground flaxseed *or* Nutri Flax

¾ cup light-flavor honey *or* maple syrup

2 tablespoons soft unsalted butter, ghee (clarified butter), *or* coconut oil

¼ to ½ cup pure water, if necessary to thin the batter

1 cup raisins *or* chopped prunes

Preheat the oven to 425°F.

Lightly oil a muffin tin or line with unbleached paper cups.

In a large bowl, combine the dry ingredients. In another large bowl, beat together the yogurt, egg, honey, and butter. Add the pure water if necessary to thin the batter. Add dry ingredients and fold in with a few quick strokes. Fold in the raisins. Fill prepared muffin tin two-thirds full.

Bake 15 to 20 minutes or until done.

Quinoa Salad

Yield: 4 to 6 servings

1 cup quinoa, uncooked

2 cups pure water

1 clove garlic, crushed or diced

½ cup diced celery

½ cup grated carrot

1 rounded teaspoon nutritional yeast (optional)

Place the quinoa in a fine-mesh sieve and rinse well with pure water. Pour quinoa in a medium saucepan and add the pure water. Bring to a boil, then immediately turn down the heat to low. Cook covered for 15 minutes or until all of the water is absorbed. If you want a warm salad, immediately mix in the rest of the ingredients. If you prefer a cold salad, let the quinoa salad cool and refrigerate for at least 1 hour before eating. For a more mellow flavor, cook the garlic with the quinoa. Toss with your favorite dressing. The *Guilt Free Indulgence* Ginger Dressing (page 229) is an excellent choice here.

Quick Chunky Tomato Sauce

Yield: 4 servings

Eating tomatoes helps protect you from free radicals by trapping them. For those who eschew grains for health reasons, I recommend adding fiber to homemade or canned soups. It is especially good in tomato or vegetable soup. You may also try adding some additional fiber (Colon Care Formula or Nutri Flax) to tomato sauce, especially if you are eating a refined pasta. Add 1 teaspoon for each 1 to 2 servings.

2 tablespoons olive oil
¼ cup onion, chopped
1 clove garlic, crushed or minced
1 jar (1 pound, 12 ounces) whole Italian-style plum
  tomatoes with juices
1 cup pure water
1 tablespoon plus 1 teaspoon Colon Care Formula *or*
  Nutri Flax
1 tablespoon fresh basil leaves, julienned, *or* 1 teaspoon dried basil leaves
1 tablespoon fresh basil leaves, torn (for garnish)
Salt and fresh ground black pepper, to taste

Heat olive oil in a medium skillet; stir in onion. Sauté over low heat until tender, about 5 minutes. Stir in garlic, and sauté 1 minute. Add tomatoes and cook over medium heat, stirring and breaking up the tomatoes with the side of a spoon until boiling. Simmer sauce uncovered until slightly thickened, about 15 minutes. Stir in the water and the Colon Care Formula or Nutri Flax. Cook for 1 to 2 minutes before adding the basil, salt, and pepper. Toss with hot pasta and garnish with remaining basil leaves. Season and serve.

Gazpacho

Yield: 4 servings of 1 cup each

Here's another tomato offering from Health Coach's Guilt Free Indulgence.

There are many varieties of this Spanish national soup, but this recipe is one of the best and certainly the healthiest. Flavored with fresh herbs, gazpacho supplies plenty of vitamin A and potassium and is wonderful served cold in the traditional way or, if you prefer, heated up. This soup does not require any cooking, and therefore it retains the vitality of its fresh ingredients and can be "whipped up" in a jiffy. Perfect for Thermos lunches and picnics.

¼ white onion, chopped

⅓ cucumber, peeled, seeded, and chopped

¼ cup green pepper, chopped

1 clove garlic (or more if desired), chopped

1 teaspoon minced fresh cilantro *or* ¼ teaspoon dried coriander

5 ripe tomatoes, unpeeled and chopped

1 (6-ounce) can organic or natural tomato juice with no additives

1 tablespoon flaxseed oil

1 tablespoon red wine vinegar *or* lemon juice

Pinch of vegetable seasoning
Dash of Tabasco sauce
4 celery stalks with leaves (use celery hearts),
    chopped
1 tablespoon chives, minced
1 tablespoon fresh basil *or* parsley leaves, minced
Celery stalks (for garnish)

Place all the ingredients except celery, chives, and basil in a blender or food processor and purée until desired consistency (smooth or chunky). Mix the purée with the chopped celery, chives, and basil. Chill and serve along with whole celery stalks in cold soup bowls garnished with herbs. Add more Tabasco sauce, garlic, or cayenne for a spicier soup.

Note: If you want to increase your fiber intake for the day, you can add 2 to 4 teaspoons of Colon Care Formula or Nutri Flax to this recipe.

Immunity Boosting Soup

Yield: 6 to 10 servings (or freeze half of the pot for later enjoyment)

The potatoes give this soup a lot of body. Try it plain or with either of the herb seasonings offered. Also, try substituting winter squash for potatoes and adding a sweet cashew nut milk (see Variation page 236).

1 onion, sliced or diced
5 to 10 cloves garlic, coarsely chopped
Sesame oil *or* water, as needed
1 bunch kale, collards, mustard greens, *or* Swiss
    chard, coarsely chopped
3 potatoes, well-scrubbed, chopped into 1-inch cubes

2 summer squash *or* zucchini, chopped
2 celery stalks, chopped
4 to 10 shiitake mushrooms, sliced
1 to 1½ quarts soup stock

In a large saucepan, sauté the onion and garlic in oil or water. You may add the other vegetables one at a time to the pan to coat them and seal in the nutrients, or you can immediately add the soup stock to the sautéed onions and garlic. My soup stock is usually the water left over from previously steamed vegetables that I keep frozen in yogurt containers until needed. I don't bother to defrost the stock. I run the container upside-down under water until the frozen mass loosens (like a homemade Popsicle). The frozen stock will melt in the cooking pot after being covered with a lid. When the stock starts to simmer you can add the rest of the vegetables.

Or do it the easy way: Cut up all of the vegetables or chop them in a food processor, add the soup stock and veggies to the pot, cover, and cook over medium heat until done (about 30 minutes). Less cooking time is needed if you use a food processor to chop your vegetables, because they will be in smaller pieces. If you use this last method of preparation, be sure to watch the pot and stir the ingredients so that the vegetables don't burn while the frozen stock is melting.

Variation: For a different flavor, substitute 1 acorn or butternut squash, skin removed and cubed, for potatoes.

Two Herb Seasonings for Potato Version of Immunity Boosting Soup

Try either of these recipes with the potato version of Immunity Boosting Soup for more potency and flavor.

1 tablespoon fresh rosemary, finely chopped *or* 1½
teaspoons dried rosemary
Salt and pepper, to taste
or
½ teaspoon dried sage
1 to 2 bay leaves
Salt and pepper, to taste

For each recipe, simply blend ingredients together and use as a topping for individual bowls of soup.

Seasoning for Winter Squash Version of Immunity Boosting Soup

If you make this soup with winter squash instead of potatoes, try this seasoning recipe.

1 teaspoon cinnamon
¼ teaspoon ground cumin
¼ teaspoon ground nutmeg or fresh grated, to taste
Salt and pepper, to taste

Blend all ingredients in a bowl and then sprinkle on top of individual bowls of soup.

Variation: To increase the anticarcinogenic effect of this variety, make a milk of 1 cup cashews by softening them in 2 cups pure water for a few hours. If you don't want to wait or don't have the time, blend cashews with enough water to make into a milky consistency. You can strain the nut meat out if you like. I prefer to leave it in and get all of the protective nutrients that I can from these sweet nuts.

Note: It is best to grind your black pepper fresh, because ground pepper that sits around oxidizes and becomes carcinogenic.

Alkaline Broth

This recipe is good nourishment during a cleanse or anytime.
Simply put all of the best vegetables you can find into a pot.

Potatoes, well-scrubbed and chopped
Zucchini, chopped
Celery, chopped
Beets, chopped
Swiss chard, chopped
Green beans, chopped
Carrots, chopped
Spinach, chopped
Parsley, chopped
Fresh or dried herbs of your choice, to taste

Place ingredients in a large pot, cover with pure water, and simmer. If you want a fresher, chunkier broth, cook only until vegetables are tender, approximately 10 minutes. Put the entire mixture into a blender or food processor and whirl until puréed.

If you favor a broth, cook the vegetables for up to 60 minutes, strain, and toss the vegetables but not the broth. Savor the broth; it's filled with nutrients. This is nice to put in a Thermos and sip throughout the day as an antidote to an acid-forming, stressful schedule.

RECIPES FOR HORMONE SUPPORT

In chapters 2 and 6, I spoke about the importance of hormone health for the elimination of toxins, and about the benefits of internal cleansing. Following are recipes based on soy products that can help your body make the hormones you need to activate your elimination systems.

Better Than Chocolate Pudding

Yield: 4 servings

> 1 package (8 ounces) firm tofu
> ⅛ to ¼ cup carob powder*
> 6 to 8 large pitted dates**
> 1 teaspoon to 1 tablespoon orange zest
> 1 teaspoon vanilla *or* anise flavoring
> Nuts or fresh fruit slices (for garnish)

Crumble the tofu into a blender or food processor. Add the carob powder. Blend at medium speed. Blend in dates, orange zest, and flavoring. For a smooth consistency, blend the mixture several times. To preserve your appliance motor, turn it off after 30 seconds, scrape the sides of the container to mix the ingredients thoroughly, and blend again. Refrigerate for 30 minutes before serving if you like your pudding chilled. Top with nuts or slices of fresh fruit.

*Note: You may need to rub the carob through a fine sieve if it is lumpy.

**Note: Take as much skin as possible off of the dates if it is easy. If not, soak dates in pure warm water in a covered container for 15 minutes before adding them to the rest of the ingredients.

Whipped "Cream," Tofu Style

Yield: 4 servings

I like this whipped cream better than dairy-style because it has more body and holds up much better when mixed with the fruit in recipes such as Fruit Parfait. It also has the advantage of nourishing your hormones without adding cholesterol to your heart, arteries, or veins.

1 package (8 ounces) firm tofu
Juice of ½ small lemon
¼ to ½ cup sweetener, to taste
¼ to 1 teaspoon vanilla, to taste

Blend all the ingredients together following the recommendations for Better Than Chocolate Pudding.

Fruit Parfait

Yield: 4 servings

Here's a chance to be creative and add variety to your diet based on the best of the season or what's available in the freezer compartment.

2 cups fresh or frozen* fruit, cut into bite-size pieces
1 cup nuts (optional)
1 recipe Whipped "Cream," Tofu Style

Spoon alternating layers of cut fruit (and nuts, if desired) with Whipped "Cream," Tofu Style in a clear bowl or parfait glass.

Variations: Instead of fruit, try 1 cup applesauce. Once I made a strawberry-rhubarb compote by mixing equal parts of fruit and cooking them over low heat for 15 minutes. I added sweetener to taste for the last 5 minutes of cooking, then let the fruit compote cool before layering with the Whipped "Cream."

Note: In the winter, you can use frozen fruit, but be sure it is well thawed before layering with the Whipped "Cream." To thaw the fruit, microwave it for up to 2 minutes or heat over a double boiler until softened.

DRINK RECIPES FOR TOTAL NUTRITIONAL SUPPORT

Fruit Smoothie

Yield: 1 to 2 servings

One of the easiest ways to get the nutrition from fresh fruit, probiotic formulas, and fiber is to add it all to a smoothie. Use a variety of ingredients to whip up a delicious, nutritious treat extraordinaire.

> 1 cup live-culture non-fat yogurt
> ⅔ cup fresh or frozen fruit
> 1 teaspoon Colon Care Formula *or* Nutri Flax
> 1 teaspoon flaxseed oil
> ¼ teaspoon Ultra Flora Plus
> 1 tablespoon Probioplex Intensive Care
> Sweetener, to taste (optional)

Place all ingredients in a blender and process until smooth.

Variations: You may also add aloe juice to heal your gut. Use 2 to 4 ounces per drink.

Another superfood that I add to my concoction is algae.

If you use brewer's yeast, bee pollen, or Metagenics PhytoComplete, you can add them to your smoothie.

Instead of yogurt, I most often use one of the Ultra Clear powders designed by Dr. Bland (mixed with pure water) to ensure that I get good nutrition to start my day.

If you're not sure how it would taste to add all of those unusual ingredients to your smoothie, start simple with one or two additives and work your way up to find the perfect brew for you. If you don't have a blender, mix all of the ingredients in a bowl and enjoy. I omit algae and the Ultra Clear products if I eat this recipe in a bowl (because in a milkshake you aren't staring at the green algae, but in a bowl . . .).

Note: If you are sensitive to dairy products, you may use nut, soy, rice, or oat milk (available in your health food store), or use more fruit and pure water.

Silly Pudding

Yield: 2 servings

I call this pudding silly because it contains psyllium husks and also because it is pretty untraditional.

> 8 ounces fruit juice
> ½ cup organic raisins, soaked in warm water for at
>   least 30 minutes
> 2 teaspoons Colon Care Formula *or* Nutri Flax
> ½ cup sliced bananas
> Pure water, as needed to create desired consistency

Shake or blend vigorously the juice, raisins, and Colon Care Formula or Nutri Flax in a glass jar or blender. Pour into a bowl and top with banana slices. The fiber will absorb all of the water and congeal to the consistency of pudding in a few minutes. If you like, add some of your favorite flavoring, such as vanilla or cinnamon, and nuts for crunch.

Mild Laxative Treats

Yield: 8 to 10 balls

> 1 pint dried fruit (such as raisins, prunes, dates, figs, or unsulfured apricots), mixed, soaked, and mashed
> 1 ounce carob powder
> 1 ounce ground licorice root
> 1 ounce slippery elm powder
> ½ cup Colon Care Formula *or* Nutri Flax
> Sweetener, to taste
> 2 ounces shredded coconut (optional)
> Shredded coconut *or* sesame seeds as needed (toasted, if desired), for rolling

In a medium bowl, mix together all ingredients except shredded coconut (or sesame seeds) for rolling. To prevent the dough from sticking to your hands, oil your hands. Roll teaspoonfuls of dough into little balls, and then roll them in the coconut or sesame seeds.

Refrigerate or freeze before serving to make the balls firm.

SUGGESTED MENUS

Breakfast

If you need to eat a low-carbohydrate diet, I recommend having a shake of Ultra Clear or Ultra Clear Plus for breakfast for an optimally balanced protein-carbohydrate-fat ratio. Just put the powder and pure water into a closed container and shake—you are ready to fly! What could be simpler? If you have chosen to add some of the probiotic formulas, try mixing up a Fruit Smoothie (page 241). This nutritive, quick breakfast will get you well nourished and supercharged to start your day.

If you prefer solid food but have little time, try a banana, apple, pear, or other fresh fruit coated with a tablespoon of sesame, almond, cashew, or sunflower butter. If you are prone to herpes outbreaks, take a 500-milligram tablet of lysine with this quick and delicious meal. Try not to eat peanuts in any form because they may have an inflammatory effect on your body—unless it is for the sheer joy of the taste of peanut sauce on your food, as in Thai food.

Or try eating like the Asians. Have chicken or fish soup with vegetables for breakfast. This is a little unusual for most Americans, but a good option for carbohydrate-intolerant individuals. This breakfast will keep your motor happily humming for many hours.

If you are able to tolerate and enjoy carbohydrates, try the recipes for Instant Hot Cereal (page 230), Blueberry Oatmeal (page 231), or Fiber Muffins (page 231). People who like this option for breakfast but don't have the desire or facility to grind the grains can cook up a big pot of grains in the evening when they have more time and store the leftovers in the refrigerator. In the morning, simply heat up some of the grains in a pot or in the microwave oven with some milk (cow's, goat's, nut, soy, rice, or oat) for a satisfying and tasty meal. You can make this savory dish even better by adding miso or soy sauce and brewer's yeast, or try spicing it up by adding cayenne or garlic. You might also try sweetening it by adding applesauce, fruit, or raisins, but be careful; many people find that eating fruit and grains together causes intestinal gas. Another variation is to add nuts, keeping in mind the same cautions about nut or seed butters that we've mentioned previously: If you are prone to herpes outbreaks, add a lysine supplement.

If you are the kind of person who does best with a light first meal, you might want to try the Antioxidant Fruit Salad (page 226) or just eat a piece of fresh fruit. Alkaline Broth (page 238) is another breakfast option to consider.

To ensure that you start your day with those health-promoting omega-3 essential fatty acids, add a teaspoon to a tablespoon (depending on your body weight and the doses you will be taking later in the day) of fresh flaxseed oil to a shake, soup, or grain mixture. Remember, never cook with fresh flaxseed oil; add the oil to a soup or grain dish after placing it in a bowl to eat.

Lunch

If you want to lose weight, lunch should be your biggest meal of the day. Having most of your calories at this meal gives you ample time to burn off excess calories with your activities of the day. A short walk—even marching in place while returning calls—after lunch sets up your metabolism to burn more effectively for hours when you do finally sit down and get to work.

For a lunch that will power you through your afternoon, try the Antioxidant Vegetable Salad (page 227) with a piece of tofu, fish, or chicken. For a tasty salad dressing, try Lemon and Garlic (page 227), Poppy Seed (page 228), Ginger (page 229), or Lemon-Orange Dressing (page 229).

For a more complex carbohydrate meal, try Quinoa Salad (page 232) with any of the dressings mentioned previously to ensure a dose of omega-3 and omega-6 essential fatty acids with your noontime meal.

Quick Chunky Tomato Sauce (page 233) on top of potatoes, cooked grains, or whole grain pasta is a welcome taste treat for lunch. If you are carbohydrate-intolerant, simply serve the sauce on top of tuna, fish, chicken, or beans.

Gazpacho (page 234) or Immunity Boosting Soup (page 235) will nourish you for a full afternoon. If you feel you need more calories for lunch, simply add a high-quality protein source or a complex carbohydrate.

If you are rushed for lunch, it is best to have a shake as described in the Breakfast section. That way you will avoid creating the toxic breakdown products of undigested food eaten under stress.

Dinner

Dinner is often the most relaxed meal of the day—a time when you can slow down and really enjoy what you are eating. Try any of the options mentioned for lunch.

Here is an opportunity to make up for what may have been lacking in your food choices during the day. Think about what you have eaten so far. Have you taken in your 30 to 60 grams of fiber for optimal health? If not, you may choose to eat a lot of vegetables for dinner and a high-fiber dessert such as Antioxidant Fruit Salad (page 226), Better Than Chocolate Pudding (page 239), Silly Pudding (page 242), or Mild Laxative Treats (page 243). Did you take in your appropriate amount of omega-3 fatty acids as described in chapter 3? If not, have one of the dressings mentioned previously on your salad, grains, or vegetables; eat fish for dinner; or at least take one or two DHA capsules (depending on your weight and what you have already taken in during the day) to allow your nervous system to recharge while you sleep.

If you have not had enough pure water during the day (at least 32 ounces) drink some as soon as you get home. If you drink it too close to bedtime, you may have to make unexpected trips to the bathroom when you would be better off dreaming.

For your intestinal health, in addition to the fiber, EFAs, and water, have you had your probiotics? Be sure to eat one of the following: yogurt, kefir, Probioplex Intensive Care, or Ultra Flora Plus.

If you have fulfilled all of these recommendations, you can go to bed knowing you have done the best you could do for yourself this day nutritionally. If you did not, then you have the option of making healthier choices tomorrow.

Bon appétit!

CHAPTER 14

SUPPLEMENTS TO SUPPORT CLEANSING

DAILY NOURISHING TEA

If you prefer doing a mild cleanse and finding your nutrients in herbal teas, I recommend Daily Nourishing Tea from Mountain Wild Herbals. The ingredients are red clover, horsetail, nettles, alfalfa, oat straw, licorice, and rose hips. These herbs are all grown organically and dried fresh (see appendix 1 for ordering information). Daily Nourishing Tea is supportive to the acid/base balance. It is gently alkalinizing, to neutralize the acid-inducing stress of our modern lives, and high in vitamins and minerals. (Its previous name was Detoxification Tea, to acknowledge its use as a gentle cleansing formula.) The ingredients (in alphabetical order) contain the following nutritional factors:

- **Alfalfa:** potassium; magnesium; iron; manganese; copper; calcium; phosphorus; vitamins A, C, D, E, K, B_1, B_{12}, and niacin

- **Horsetail:** calcium, silica, bioflavonoids, iron, magnesium
- **Licorice:** phosphorus, iron, magnesium
- **Nettles:** calcium; phosphorus; potassium; iron; silica; copper; sulfur; and vitamins A, C, D, and K
- **Oat straw:** magnesium, steroidal saponins (stabilize blood sugar), and calcium (and synergistic minerals and vitamins that aid calcium absorption); reduces cholesterol and risk of heart disease; nourishes central nervous system
- **Red clover:** B-complex vitamins, vitamin C, calcium
- **Rose hips:** vitamin C

In tea form, the nutrients are easy to assimilate because they are more like a food. They smell delicious and are easy to make. In my office, we brew up a pot in the morning and keep it out in a thermal teapot for our staff, clients, and patients.

PROBIOTIC FORMULAS

Probiotics are a class of nutrients that supply and encourage health-promoting bacteria in your intestines. They include, but are not limited to, mother's milk, fiber acidophilus, bifidobacteria, fructo-oligosaccharides (FOSs), and inulin (from dandelion), which can be found in Yerba Prima's Herbal Guard, a component of the Men's Rebuild and Women's Renew programs (discussed in chapter 9) and the Metagenics products Ultra Clear Sustain, Ultra Flora Plus, and Probioplex Intensive Care. As you have learned in previous chapters, healthy intestines support your good health by promoting the formation of B-vitamins, immune boosters, and anticarcinogenic substances. You may use probiotics every day—not only when you cleanse—to improve your health and well-being.

When choosing a probiotic formula to recommend to my patients, I considered four factors:

- **Stomach acid and bile resistance:** Will the friendly bacteria live through the digestive process? Most strains of acidophilus get broken down before they even enter the large intestine.
- **Ability to colonize:** Will they be able to attach to the bowel wall then colonize and multiply? To improve bowel health for a longer period of time than it takes to move through the colon, the bacteria must be able to set up residence on the bowel wall. Most acidophilus strains are unable to do this.
- **Refrigeration:** Is the product refrigerated? The beneficial bugs need a cool environment in the outside world to stay alive. If the product is on the shelf in the health food store or was not shipped in a refrigerated package, it is probably useless.
- **Independent laboratory assays:** Will the supplier provide you with an independent laboratory analysis of their product? Each batch of Metagenics probiotic formulas has been assayed by a lab independent of Metagenics to assure the quantity and viability of the friendly bacteria that are claimed to be in the bottle.
- The NCFM (North Carolina Food and Microbiology) strain of acidophilus meets all criteria. Metagenics/Ethical Nutrients holds the exclusive right to use the NCFM strain.

A study by Vicki L. Hughes, M.T., and Sharon L. Hilier, Ph.D., of the Department of Obstetrics and Gynecology,

University of Washington, Seattle, looked at the effect of acidophilus products on vaginitis, which causes itching and discharge from the vagina. As a preliminary step, they analyzed approximately 20 different acidophilus products to find the best one to use in their study. Only one product had any viable, living acidophilus in it. The rest of the products not only did not have the good guys in the bottle, they included pathogenic (disease-producing) bacteria. Although the one product contained live acidophilus cultures, we do not know whether it could hold up to the rigorous standards required of Ultra Flora Plus, the Metagenics product that I recommend. Ultra Flora Plus is available at nutritionally minded doctors' offices, in regular and dairy-free forms (see appendix 1 for contact information).

Cultured milk products such as yogurt may also contain beneficial live cultures of what we affectionately call in our office "bif and doph"—the friendly bacteria. However, because of the problem with bovine somatotropic hormone (BSH—a potential carcinogen; see chapter 4) being used by commercial dairies to increase milk yields, I recommend getting yogurt made from the milk of organically raised cows. You can generally find organically made yogurt in your health food store. If that is not possible, the next best choice is nonfat yogurt from your supermarket; hormone residue lives in the fat portion of milk products, so by eliminating the fat, you are better protected. Here is another label-reading opportunity: Make sure the label states that the product contains live cultures. Some companies heat yogurt after it is packed, which destroys our little friends.

Another probiotic formula, Probioplex Intensive Care by Metagenics, combines a number of nutritional components that nourish friendly bacteria and obliterate harmful microbes. Nourishment is provided from FOSs (discussed at length in chapter 9), maltodexetrin, and lecithin. A team of nutrients (concentrated activated globulin whey, lactoferrin, and lactoperoxidase) coats, starves, and kills the "bad guys." In a process called opsonization, the activated globulin coats the pathogens and alerts your immune system cells to their presence. In the colon, lactoferrin binds to iron, a food source for pathogenic microorganisms, thus depriving the microorganisms of nourishment (your body receives all the iron it needs by absorption higher up in your small intestines). Finally, lactoperoxidase kills the bad guys by damaging their cell walls. This team of nutrients acts selectively against harmful microbes and for the health and proliferation of the good guys. People sensitive to dairy products may not be able to tolerate this product (for more information, see appendix 1).

SUPPORT FOR A HEALTHY INTESTINAL ENVIRONMENT FOR MICROBES

The gastrointestinal tract serves as a critical immune and physical barrier between what you take in from the outside world in the form of food and drink and your body's cells. A healthy intestinal environment for microbes (the "good bugs" in your intestines) plays a critical role in supporting these functions. Metagenics has designed a protocol for nutritional support of your intestinal tract. The protocol starts with the fundamentals of a healthy environment, adds digestive support, then helps normalize a dysfunctional bowel with aggressive herbal support and complementary care. The fundamental support is provided by Ultra Flora Plus (mentioned previously).

Digestive support comes in the form of digestive enzymes. Remember the adage, "You are what you eat?" As stated previously, you are what you absorb. Even if you eat the finest food, if you are not absorbing the nutrients from it, you will not feel your best. Metagenics digestive support consists of broad-spectrum enzymes, a raw pancreatic enzyme concentrate, and/or stomach acidifiers. SpectraZyme supplies a broad spectrum of non-animal-derived enzymes that support digestive function. Metagest contains betaine hydrochloride (HCL), combined with the proteolytic enzyme pepsin and gentian root, an herbal bitter traditionally used to support digestion. Metagest supports the first major phase of digestion. If your stomach is not acidic enough, the pancreas will not have enough stimulation to release its alkaline enzymes, leaving your bowel in a compromised state.

Azeo-Pangen is a comprehensive enzyme complex that provides support for the second major phase of digestive function by featuring a raw pancreatic enzyme concentrate.

Aggressive support comes in the form of carefully formulated herbal formulas: a concentrated garlic compound and another probiotic formula. CandiBactin-AR is a concentrated blend of essential oils and herbal extracts from the aromatic mint family in a formula designed to support a healthy balance of microbes in the intestines. The formula features extracts of red thyme oil and basil, traditionally used to harmonize gastrointestinal and respiratory function. The relationship between the health of these two organ systems is well recognized in traditional health practices. In turn, the health of your gut and your lungs is essential for a strong immune system. The intestinal mucosa is an integral part of the immune system, and maintaining a healthy microbial balance there supports the health and function of all tissues and organs in the body. The ancient healing systems of Asia, Europe, and North and South America considered the mint family invigorating and stimulating. This pungent plant family is one of the most popular worldwide for supporting digestive health and microbial balance in the intestines while maintaining a healthy respiratory system.

CandiBactin-BR features 400 milligrams of berberine sulfate, purified from berberis root and standardized to berberine. Berberine, a natural substance that supports immune function and encourages the body to purge unwanted compounds, has been investigated in clinical trials.[1,2] Herbal bitters have traditionally been used for their purgative qualities to soothe the stomach, stimulate digestive secretions, and harmonize the action of the liver and gall bladder. Today, plant chemists have profiled "bitter principals" as possessing varied chemical structures and actions. These principals, which include berberine, alkaloids, flavonoids, and anthroquinones, are representative of the various kinds of phytochemical families that exert a profound clearing and antioxidant effect within the body, and produce the herbs' bitter taste. Drawing on both contemporary research and the traditional Chinese and Ayurvedic systems, Candi-Bactin-BR is designed to participate in the maintenance of healthy microbial balance in the intestines and the purgative functions of the gallbladder, liver, and urinary tract. The chief plants and traditional Chinese decoction in this unique formula possess multiple modes of action and harmonize the systems that support elimination.[3,4]

Ultra Parex is a powerful combination of wormwood, ginger, and sour plum, herbs traditionally used to support a healthy microbial environment and to stimulate the cathartic (purgative, stimulating evacuation, especially of the bowels) action of the digestive and eliminatory organs. Traditional Asian diets include bitter, sour, and pungent foods such as ginger and plum. These foods have been found to contain phytochemicals that contribute to balanced gut ecology while harmonizing stomach, gallbladder, and intestinal function. Ultra Parex builds upon the action of the CandiBactin products and makes an excellent travel companion and accompaniment to raw fish dishes and other unique cuisines.

SuperGarlic 6000 is a super-concentrated garlic supplement that is guaranteed to supply 6,000 micrograms of allicin and other naturally occurring health-supporting components of garlic in each tablet. Garlic has a long history of traditional use as a support for the immune system and in maintaining a healthful microbial balance.

Probioplex Intensive Care is described earlier in this chapter.

Complementary Care comes in the form of UltraInflamX and Glutagenics. UltraInflamX, a pleasant tasting, easily digested, low-allergenic powdered beverage mix, is a nutritionally diverse medical food designed to provide targeted nutritional support for patients with chronic inflammatory conditions. UltraInflamX features a unique blend of vitamins, minerals, amino acids, bioflavonoids, and the phytonutrients rutin, curcumin, and quercetin to nutritionally support essential fatty acid metabolism; detoxification; gastrointestinal mucosa integrity; and the reduction of damage from free radicals, electrically charged particles from pollution, and synthetic chemicals.

A healthy intestinal lining is essential for proper digestion, immune function, liver function, and overall health, primarily through its role as a barrier—preventing the absorption of unwanted molecules into your circulation. Unfortunately, the intestinal lining is vulnerable to a variety of insults, such as poor diet, caffeine and alcohol consumption, and use of non-steroidal anti-inflammatory drugs (NSAIDs; such as aspirin and ibuprofen). It's important to provide support for this delicate mucosal environment to ensure its optimal integrity and function. Glutagenics contains a synergistic blend of ingredients that help promote a healthy intestinal lining.

Glutagenics contains three key ingredients: glutamine, deglycyrrhizinized licorice (DGL), and aloe. Glutamine serves as a fuel for the rapidly dividing cells of the intestinal mucosa and immune system. It enhances the function of the intestinal barrier and it transports as much as 40 percent of whole-blood nitrogen. These properties make glutamine essential for maintaining the integrity of the intestinal mucosa, promoting an optimal immune response, and supporting muscle recovery as an anticatabolic nutrient. DGL is processed to remove glycyrrhizinic acid to eliminate the potential risk of side effects associated with licorice consumption, and a premium extract of aloe leaf is standardized to 50 percent polysaccharides with the bitter principles removed to prevent the laxative effect. This form of licorice has been used in Europe for many years for its supportive effects on the gastric mucosa. DGL enhances the resistance of the gastric mucosa against the eroding effects of bile, stimulates proliferation of the gastric epithelial cells, and enhances mucous production and secretion.

Aloe is traditionally used to enhance tissue synthesis and promote healthy mucous membranes of the intestinal lining. The active principals, acemannan and mannose, support balanced immune function. In addition, aloe is thought to bind to receptor sites in the gut, enhancing its barrier function.

The activity of each ingredient in Metagenics products is confirmed by independent laboratory analysis prior to inclusion in their formulas and standardized to ensure herbal quality and activity.

FREE RADICALS AND OXIDATIVE STRESS

Free radicals are highly reactive molecules, originating from internal and external pollution, that can cause tissue damage by reacting with fatty acids in your cell membranes, portions of your DNA, and critical bonds in your protein structures (joints, muscles, organs, glands, and so on). To visualize the damage that free radicals can do, think about what exposure to air does to a cut apple or to untreated metal: Apples turn brown and taste bad, and metal rusts. Free radicals have been implicated in the development of more than 50 diseases, including allergies, fibromyalgia, chronic fatigue, arthritis and other inflammatory diseases; neurological diseases; kidney disease; cataracts; bowel disease; lung dysfunction; drug reactions; skin problems; and aging. Heart disease and cancer are strongly associated with free radical damage. More and more studies are linking low dietary intake of antioxidants to an increased risk of heart disease. Antioxidants are nutrients that bind to toxins and biochemically alter their chemical structure. Conversely, a reduction of cancer risk is associated with diets high in antioxidants such as vitamin C. Free radicals cause damage to your cells, resulting in internal pollution in your body.

Solutions to Free Radical Stress

Saturate your environment with negative ions, which help trap positively charged pollution particles. You can purchase negative ion generators, but they tend to make a big black spot on surfaces near where they work because they attract soot and pollution particles. Some newer models have a foam collar that is intended to catch the pollution particles so that they don't collect on your walls and furniture, but they are not completely effective.

You can also get negative ions for free; they are present in the mist of running water, among other things. A friend in chiropractic school had a solution for whatever ailed you: Take a shower. Sometimes she took three showers a day. Once I learned about the high concentration of negative ions in shower spray, I better understood her panacea. A shower is especially good if you have a water filter in place (see appendix 1 for information on where you can find a water filter).

Other suggestions for increasing your "happy particle" stream include taking a walk at night (negative ions are more highly concentrated in the night air), spending time with plants (pointed plant leaves concentrate negative ions), and performing yogic breathing exercises. To do the latter, breathe through one nostril at a time by closing the other nostril with your thumb or middle finger.

Oxidative Stress

Oxidative stress is the cellular damage caused by free radicals. Antioxidant supplements and antioxidant foods trap these free radicals, protecting your cells and improving the outcome of your cleansing programs (for more on antioxidant foods, see chapter 13). Are you at risk for oxidative stress? See the Oxidative Stress Questionnaire in appendix 4 to find out. A yes answer to any of these questions may mean that you are not meeting your antioxidant needs and thus are vulnerable to the damage that free radicals can cause. If you do have oxidative stress, see appendix 1 to learn about the types of nutrients that quench free radicals.

CHAPTER 15

PRACTICES THAT COMPLEMENT CLEANSING

Several techniques can complement and enhance an internal cleansing program. They encourage a more active cleansing and prevent the possibility of any severe reactions to the cleansing. I feel that the most important of these techniques are conscious relaxation; drinking water; exercise; dry skin brushing; and supplementing your diet with aloe vera, bentonite, and probiotics (discussed in chapters 13 and 14).

We have seen that the world in which we live places an amazing burden on the natural cleansing systems of our bodies. If you do not assist your cleansing systems in removing the waste your cells are swimming in every day, you may be subject to degenerative diseases that could rob you of a happy, healthy life. But as you incorporate cleansing practices into your lifestyle, you will receive many other benefits of good health.

EVALUATE THE HEALTH IMPACT OF YOUR PRIORITIES

The Greek philosopher Epictetus said, "Men are disturbed not by things, but by the view they take of them." Our minds can be our greatest ally, but also our greatest enemy. It is important to determine what role your thoughts, emotions, and beliefs actually play with respect to your health.

There are no shortcuts to health any more than there are to raising healthy crops or animals. To be in good health, you must first be clear about how much you value your health. Then you must live a life of integrity in alignment with the timeless, unchanging laws and principles that govern health. A beneficial exercise is to pause and write down what you value in life and what those things mean to you. Take your time. Perhaps revisit what you have written a day or two later. Are you making time for what you value in your life? If not, you will benefit by spending half an hour a week to shape your schedule around what is important before you get swallowed by the river of life. Steven Covey's *First Things First* (see Bibliography) is a good guide to life management.

LOSE TOXIC-LADEN FAT

One of the most common benefits reported by those who have done internal cleansing is that they seem to lose weight without even trying. If you follow a careful cleansing program such as I've described, you lose weight because you are losing fat. As you have read, fat is the storage place for toxins in your body. When you lose fat, you are helping to decrease your toxic load. Much of the weight loss comes from the stomach and waistline, where a distended colon has given the appearance of fat. Many people who have dieted for years, and have lost weight in all portions of their bodies except the stubborn stomach region, find that these protrusions disappear through cleansing. If you have been unable to lose that thick area around your middle, it may not be due solely to overeating as much as to a desperate need to cleanse your intestines.

In addition, cleansing the intestinal tract will enable your body's systems to work more efficiently so that you will absorb more nutrients from the foods you eat. Many times, people eat too much because their body is not being nutritionally satisfied from the foods they eat. This is caused not only by eating the wrong foods but also by a sluggish, blocked system that is unable to absorb nutrients. Both a high-fiber diet and a thorough cleansing will greatly enhance nutrient absorption and reduce the tendency to be addicted to foods that have no nutritional value.

Reducing the volume of carbohydrates that you eat in the form of grains, bread, pasta, crackers, waffles, pancakes, and so on may also help you get rid of unwanted fat. A long-term patient of mine has been trying to lose that last 5 pounds ever since she had her children, more than 20 years ago, but whatever she tried failed. Finally, she took my advice and eliminated almost all grains and grain products from her diet. She is now happy to show me her flat stomach and celebrate losing those last 5 pounds.

Dr. Stephen T. Chang, a Chinese medical specialist and Taoist Master, teaches the Crane Exercise, an energetic practice to improve the health of your gastrointestinal system and abdominal organs (kidneys, adrenals, pancreas, bladder, and reproductive organs). I came across this helpful practice in the 1980s in his now out-of-print booklet, *How to Rub Your Stomach Away: The Crane Exercise*. A more recent book by Dr. Chang, which includes the Crane Exercise in more detail, is *The Complete System of Self-Healing: Internal Exercises*.

The Crane Exercise has two components, physical and energetic. The physical component is a slow circular rubbing motion. The energetic component is imagining or visualizing heat and energy filling the lower part of your body. This exercise is most beneficial when performed twice a day (or more if you like) for only 2 minutes each time, while lying on your back. The best times are before you get out of bed in the morning and before you go to sleep at night.

The rubbing motion begins at the navel and proceeds in increasingly large spirals in a clockwise direction (from right to left) using the hand that you write with. Once you have reached the limits of your lower rib cage and pubic bone, reverse the spiral, proceeding in a counterclockwise direction (from left to right) in gradually smaller spirals until you are back at your navel. While you move your hand, visualize heat or energy warming and brightening your whole abdomen. Imagine blockages in your intestines and organs breaking up and passing out of your body. Imagine excess fat cells melting away.

Unlike liposuction, you won't see immediate results, *but* you won't have to deal with the pain or the expense of that procedure either. And can you imagine how good you will feel devoting some early-morning and late-night time to your own healing? I know my body likes it! Patience and persistence are the keys to success here. After all, you live with your body your whole lifetime. Doesn't it makes sense that your body will thrive if you give it loving attention?

EXERCISE TO STIMULATE THE CLEANSING PROCESS

In addition to a proper diet, the value of regular exercise cannot be overstated. Remember how toxins are stored primarily in the fatty tissue of your body? By mobilizing this toxic fat through exercise, deep breathing, sweating, and drinking lots of water, you will rid your body of this reservoir of harmful substances. Our bodies are designed for movement, and in our increasingly sedentary lives it is most important to incorporate some consistent physical activity into our schedules. If you are following the type of diet recommended in this book—high in fruits and vegetables, low in animal fats, and with the proper proportions of essential fatty acids and healthy protein—you will be able to reduce the non-beneficial fat stored in your cells to recreate a healthier you with added exercise.

First, let's take a look at the benefits of exercise; then, we'll examine some ways to fit more activity into your busy schedule.

1. Exercise strengthens and tones the muscles of the body, including those in your gastrointestinal tract. It helps to stimulate a sluggish bowel. If you are prone to constipation, exercise will help increase the activity of your bowel, making you a much more efficient eliminator of metabolic waste products.

2. Exercise increases circulation and perspiration. Your skin is your largest organ of elimination. When you sweat, toxins that are circulating in your blood and lymph and stored in the subcutaneous layers of your skin are released through your

pores, assisting your body's cleansing process and strengthening your immune system.

3. Exercise strengthens your lungs' ability to transport oxygen to your heart and to carry carbon dioxide and waste away from it.

4. Exercise increases lymphatic circulation, which supports the excretion of waste from your cells.

5. A regular exercise program greatly reduces the effects of stress and increases self-esteem. Chemicals of stress that accumulate in your system can be metabolized more efficiently when you exercise. Have you ever noticed how much better you feel after taking a walk if something is troubling you? Part of the transformation comes from the breakdown of stress hormones that have stayed lodged in your body tissues just waiting for release.

6. Exercise raises your metabolic rate to more efficiently use the calories you take in, especially if you exercise within one half-hour of eating.

7. Consistently following an exercise program makes you feel more balanced, healthier, stronger, and more self-confident.

Regular exercise strengthens all of your body's systems, enabling you to function optimally. The natural cleansing and elimination systems that are so valuable to you in preventing the buildup of toxic waste will be made stronger and more efficient by physical activity. Steven Blair, M.D., has this to say about exercise in his book, *Living with Exercise:* "A good exercise prescription for the thirty to fifty million mostly sedentary and unfit Americans is 'turn off the television, get off your fanny, go out the door, and move around a bit.' We have learned from research that it often doesn't matter what you do. Any activity that increases your metabolic rate and burns more calories provides benefits." Whether you choose an aerobic activity (one that raises your heart rate significantly) or a series of stretching exercises, what is most important is consistency. It is said that if you maintain an exercise program for 6 months, it will become a healthy habit for life. Even a brisk walk taken for 10 minutes daily will benefit you in many ways. Here's a wonderful quote about exercise from Edward Stanley, the Earl of Derby, in 1873: "Those who think they have not time for bodily exercise will sooner or later have to find time for illness."

It is never too late to begin an exercise program. William Evans, Ph.D., chief of the Human Physiology Laboratory at Tufts University, Human Nutrition Research Center on Aging, has witnessed a 90-year-old patient become stronger than a 50-year-old through consistent exercise. The center's oldest exerciser is 100 years of age. One of my male patients, 55 years old, belongs to a softball team called the "Seniors." Their ages range from 50 to 70. When you reach 70 in their league, you join the "Creakers" team of men who are from 70 to 90 years of age.

How do you fit more activity into a busy but largely sedentary lifestyle? You have heard this before: Park your car a block away from where you are going so that you get more leg work on your way to and from your errands. If you live in an area with public transportation, consider taking it once in a while; generally there is some extra walking getting back and forth between stations or bus stops. Take the stairs instead of the elevator, if not the whole way, at least for a landing or two. Stand up when you are talking on the telephone; it will make your voice stronger and give you the opportunity to stretch or move your legs. To multiply the effect on your metabolic activity, gently march or step in place while talking.

While standing, you might also take the opportunity to do some pliés (pronounced "plee-AZE"), as they are called in the dance world: Keeping your back straight, place your feet a comfortable distance apart, bend your knees and lower your torso straight down a comfortable distance, then rise up by straightening your legs, and repeat. This exercise has the benefit of increasing your circulation. I remember waiting at 7:00 A.M. for my chiropractic licensing board exam to begin. A friend and I were taking the boards at the same time. We had gotten lost on the way to the exam, so we were pretty stressed out. When the examiners came parading past, I started to feel faint. Pliés saved me from passing out that day. Bending my knees and straightening them helped to get more blood moving up into my head. Pliés can even boost your performance on the job by helping you think more clearly while replacing that afternoon cup of toxic coffee.

If you have stairs at home, try walking up and down them a couple of times after eating; it will help combat that after-meal brain fog that too often brings your energy down. Or just try dancing. One of my favorite ways to exercise is to put on James Brown's *Gravity* CD and let loose! Even if you don't have music, you can make music with the rhythmic movement of your body. Here's a chance to let the kid in you out and have more fun—a great antidote for the complexity and seriousness of life. I have a lot of fun standing outside my car and stretching at gas stations when my tank is filling. Sometimes I even use the paper receptacles to stretch out my hamstrings. (Be sure to watch out for cars while engaging in your gas-station stretch routine.) While on an airplane, I always go to the open area adjacent to the movie screen and do some stretching. That raises some eyebrows, but I also notice that my stretching sets an example for other people to get off their duffs to stretch or just walk around. Some don't bother to get up but stretch in their seats anyway.

One of my dear friends has lived for a couple of years in China. She reports that people are much more active there. They do Tai Chi in the parks, massage reflex points on their bodies and faces, and walk and ride bicycles much more than we do in this country. Why not be the first to start a revolution in your office, home, or town? Bob Anderson has written some great books on stretching. He has gone so far as to make up a sheet of exercises that can be done right at your desk to ease the monotony of minuscule motions that one performs while in an office setting (see appendix 1 for more information).

Conversely, if you are the kind of person who does a lot of physical work on the job, you probably need to stretch more than you need to strengthen your muscles. Your local college or YMCA/YWCA probably has some stretch or yoga classes that would benefit you—or buy one of the many stretching videos that are on the market and use it.

Therein lies the key, doesn't it? Make the time to just do it! Working with your schedule is essential here. Steven Covey encourages us to decide what we value in our lives and then to make time for what we value by putting those things into our schedule before anything else. Did you know that in our country the most successful people and businesses spend up to 60 percent of their time planning? Plan for success this time. Either make a time in your day that is sacred—that you devote to taking good care of yourself with some type of movement—or just commit to being more active in general. Write down your successes in the area of increased movement or exercise, and celebrate. You can do it!

TAKE A BATH AND SWEAT IT OUT

If you are unable to exercise to a level that makes you sweat, you can enjoy the benefits of sweating by taking a sauna, steam bath, hot tub, or hot bath. One of my best suggestions for my patients who are sore or achy and complaining of stiff muscles as a result of toxic buildup is to take a bath with Epsom salts. Magnesium and sulfur are the main ingredients of Epsom salts. Magnesium is great for relaxing tight, sore, and tired muscles. It helps carry calcium into your muscle cells to relax them and helps your cells to get rid of toxins. (You may also take a magnesium supplement to relax your muscles if you cannot take baths. Magnesium glycinate is preferred because it is gentle to your digestive tract; other forms of magnesium can cause diarrhea. Magnesium glycinate is made and distributed by Metagenics and is available through doctor's offices.) Sulfur is one of the main ingredients in healthy joints. Therefore, Epsom salts help both your muscles and your joints, creating a strong and healthy musculoskeletal system.

Soaking in hot water, in and of itself, has a relaxing effect on your body, mind, and soul, but you can enhance that effect by putting essential oils into your bath. Only a little is needed, because the oil will disperse in the water.

Pine is said to help sore muscles and joints, and lavender is said to soothe and calm your nervous system. If you stay in the room while the tub fills, you will have the added benefit of a negative ion bath. Filter your water if possible.

BREATHE DEEPLY TO REPLACE BAD AIR WITH GOOD

Air is our first necessity for continued life. Some accomplished yogis and pearl divers are able to hold their breath or suspend overt signs of breathing for extended periods; however, the average person has no such skills. The human brain dies after being deprived of oxygen for 1 to 2 minutes.

There are ways to expand your breathing repertoire that will increase your health. Deep breathing helps exchange the "good" air for the "bad" air. Some benefits of deep breathing include the following:

- The relaxation response is enhanced when you breathe deeply. Breathing deeply helps you get out of your ever-active mind and settle into your "belly brain." In your abdomen and heart as well as in your brain, "happy hormones" are produced. Deep breathing supports their production, creating an all-over relaxation response. When you are relaxed, your body works better and life seems to go better, too. Be careful, however; you may hyperventilate and feel dizzy if you neglect to expand your whole torso all the way down to your pubic bone with each breath.

- Deep breathing can help normalize the pH in your body and support metabolic function. It helps calm the spirit and soothe the soul. It will quickly take you out of a sympathetic nervous system "fight-or-flight" alarm state and reduce the stress you are feeling in the moment.

- Deep breathing may help prevent lung cancer. The apex, or top part, of the lungs that sits above your collarbone is the most common site of lung cancer. Some lung cancer may begin here because people usually take shallow breaths that don't expand this area. Because air is not exchanged there, the area becomes a collection spot for particulate matter (such as pollution) from the air. Think of that un-used space behind your furniture or under your bed. It's exposed to air but without much circula-tion. Unless you get in there regularly to clean it out, that space harbors all kinds of dust, pollution, molds, and insects. The same thing can happen with your upper lungs.

Many excellent resources are available in the area of breath work. Yoga classes often help you focus on breathing techniques; guided relaxation audiotapes direct you to breathe deeply and slowly; and a number of self-help books have been published on this topic. (See appendix 1 for more information.)

REDUCE TOXINS WITH CHIROPRACTIC CARE

Injury from microtrauma (e.g., working at a computer for long hours at a time) or macrotrauma (e.g., a fall, an auto accident, or some other kind of structural stress) causes an accumulation of tissue-damaging toxins in your body. Studies done around the world have shown the benefits of chiropractic care in reducing or eliminating these toxic by-products of injury that lead to stiffness and pain. In New Zealand and Canada, government economists who studied the issue recommended that people with back pain see a chiropractor first so that they would be able to go back to work faster and save their governments millions of dollars. In the United States, the Agency for Health Care Policy and Research (AHCPR), a government organization, found that adjustments to the spine (performed 97 percent of the time by chiropractors) worked better at reducing uncomplicated low back pain and headache than standard medical care, including drugs and surgery.

But, as before, the most important criterion for success in internal cleansing is you, the public's response. And that information is available in terms of patient satisfaction surveys. Several studies have shown that patients are more satisfied with chiropractic care than with medical care. And what about our senior citizens? If something can help our grandparents and aging relatives enjoy a greater level of health and vitality, would it be worth checking out for yourself? *Topics in Clinical Chiropractic* published a study that showed that elderly chiropractic patients reported better overall health, had fewer chronic conditions, spent fewer days in nursing homes and hospitals, were more mobile in their communities, and were more likely to report strenuous levels of exercise than non-chiropractic patients. In short, elderly chiropractic patients were stronger and less toxic than those who did not receive chiropractic adjustments. In fact, 87 percent of chiropractic patients described their health status as good to excellent, whereas only 68 percent of non-chiropractic patients made the same claim.

Chiropractic has become a centenarian. The practice of chiropractic celebrated its 100th anniversary in September 1996. Chiropractic comprises many techniques, but all of them begin with the perspective of removing the interference in your nervous system to allow your internal healing abilities to shine brightly. One recent study that I particularly love describes the effect of chiropractic adjustments on the immune system. The study, performed at the National College of Chiropractic, measured white blood cell activity before and after spinal adjustment. When white blood cells go into action to defend against foreign invaders, they increase their oxygen uptake, as measured by an increase in luminescence (light) in the blood sample. What this means is that chiropractic adjustments help to turn on your healing light.

BRUSH YOUR SKIN

The value of dry skin brushing has been known for centuries. The Finns and Russians used and still use birch twigs to open their pores and stimulate circulation before a steam bath or sauna. The Turks used and continue to use coarse towels to rub dead skin off their body before and after the bath.

As the largest eliminative organ, the skin plays a vital role in ridding your body of toxins and impurities that are potential sources of illness. It has been estimated that the skin eliminates more than 1 pound of waste per day. For this reason, daily skin brushing is an excellent complement to an internal cleansing program.

Dry skin brushing is one of the best ways to cleanse the skin without removing the protective mantle of acid and oils. Daily skin brushing removes the top layer of dead skin, with its buildup of dirt and acid, and deeply cleanses your pores.

Skin brushing is also one of the most powerful ways to cleanse your lymphatic system. Waste material is carried away from the cells by the blood and the lymph. Skin brushing stimulates the release of this material from the cells near the surface of your skin.

In addition, dry skin brushing stimulates the sweat glands and increases blood circulation to underlying organs and tissues of the body. These days, a sedentary lifestyle, a general lack of exercise, and the use of antiperspirants keep people from sweating enough. As a result, toxins and metabolic waste products become trapped in the body instead of being released through sweat. Skin brushing opens up the pores, allowing your body to breathe and thus enhancing proper function of your organs.

Skin brushing has also been a beauty aid of men and women for ages. Removing the top layer of dead skin and stimulating blood circulation are essential for maintaining youthful, glowing, supple skin. Loss of excess weight and cellulite is an added benefit reported by a beauty salon owner in Santa Barbara, California: "I use skin brushing as part of my weight-loss and body shaping program. Skin brushing increases circulation, which helps to draw out the stored waste and toxins which often result in cellulite buildup. People tend to lose weight faster and more evenly over the entire body when skin brushing is included in their weight loss program."

How to Brush Your Skin

First, acquire an all-natural vegetable-fiber brush from your health food store (synthetic fibers will irritate your skin). A long handle is helpful for reaching your back and other less accessible surfaces of your body.

The best time to brush is before taking a shower or bath. Brushing dry skin is important, as sagging may occur if your skin or the brush is wet. Begin brushing with one-stroke movements. Brush from the outermost points—your feet and hands—toward the center of your body. Brush across your upper back and down the front and back of your torso. Cover the entire surface of the skin only once. A slight flush is normal due to increased circulation, but if your skin turns red, you may be brushing too hard.

For your face, use a softer brush or leave it alone because the blood vessels there are nearer the surface of your skin and can be broken if brushed too hard. If you do brush your face, begin in the center and stroke outward, then up the sides of your face and neck.

The total process takes only about 3 minutes. When you are finished, jump into your bath or shower and enjoy. You will feel an invigorating, tingling sensation over your entire body.

Relax and Rest to Support Your Cleansing

Negative thoughts, moods, and emotions create toxins within your body, and excess stress promotes an overgrowth of pathogenic microorganisms, which subsequently causes a buildup of toxic by-products in your intestines. Creating "healing intervals,"—times in which you "stop to smell the roses," so to speak—is vital to your ability to cleanse and heal. William Penn, founder of the state of Pennsylvania, said, "True silence is the rest of the mind; it is to the spirit what sleep is to the body: nourishment and refreshment." In questionnaires I use with my patients, I ask them how much time they spend resting during their day and how they spend their "resting" time. Often they cite watching TV as their rest time. But television watching is not the kind of healing, restorative relaxation to which I refer.

My favorite definitions of "rest" from *Webster's Dictionary* are "peace of mind or spirit" and "to be free from anxiety or disturbance." Because we are all unique individuals, we will find our peace of mind and freedom from anxiety in different ways. Currently, I most enjoy sitting on the edge of my bed, closing my eyes, placing a smile on my face, and focusing on a state of joy. When my attention drifts, I gently bring my focus back to the state of bliss that awaits me. Enjoying the beauty of nature also quickly restores my soul. When I was 22, sitting calmly made me feel agitated, so I took an "LSD" (a "long slow distance" run) or I did katas that I had learned in my karate classes. Here are some other recommendations for rest:

- Take a bath or soak in a hot tub. If you add 1 cup of Epsom salts and 1 cup of baking soda, or 2 cups of either alone, you will have the added benefit of reducing acid accumulation, which makes your muscles ache. The magnesium and sulfur in Epsom salts help your cells expel toxins and nourish your joints, respectively.
- Smile and allow the smile to wash over your entire face and body. (I explain this technique in further detail later in this chapter.)
- Take a deep breath.
- Adopt an attitude of gratitude—pause for a moment to reflect on what you are grateful for in your life, especially for your commitment to healing.

- Smell a fragrant flower.
- Hum or sing a song in your shower or in your car where no one else is listening—or, if you have a good voice, let others enjoy your singing out loud.
- Stretch your arms and legs.
- Scrunch up your face and wiggle your mouth around, then take a deep breath and sigh. Take a tip from Linus in *Classic Peanuts:* Quoting from the Bible, Romans chapter 8, he says, "Likewise the spirit helps us in our weakness; for we do not know how to pray as we ought, but the spirit him/herself intercedes for us with sighs too deep for words."
- Try to wiggle your ears.
- Dance or sway to music.
- Laugh for no reason.

Norman Cousins, who overcame a life-threatening disease by laughing at Marx Brothers movies and taking lots of vitamin C, says, "Laughter is inner jogging." The possibilities are endless. Here's another suggestion I read about in my Sunday paper: Pet a chicken. The December 1, 1996, issue of the *San Francisco Examiner* had this headline: "Chickens' new job: Lifting seniors' spirits. Saved from frying pan, birds become traveling therapists." Darrian Lundy of Green Acres farms brings her two chickens, Chickadee and Spock, to a center for older folks. "It gets people talking who haven't talked all week and generally raises their spirits," she said.

Using self-help techniques can enhance the quality of your health and your life. Your thoughts and emotions are energetic and biochemical. They have a significant effect on your health and on your relationships with others. If you dwell on worry and fear because of a past pain you experi-

enced in some part of your body, heart, or mind, you will re-
inforce your pain. If you do nothing to transform that worry
and fear, your being will store that negativity, and you may
end up with or aggravate a degenerative condition. Choose
to send love and happiness to your entire being—mind,
body, and soul—and you will enjoy greater health. Pursuing
health will be joyous work if you focus your awareness and
heart on the task.

Why don't you take a moment now to jot down some
ways of relaxing that you would enjoy? Pull your list out
and try one the next time you are exceeding your health limits. Here's some advice from Leonardo da Vinci, painter, ar-
chitect, and inventor: "Every now and then go away, even
briefly; have a little relaxation, for when you come back to
your work your judgment will be surer; since to remain constantly at work will cause you to lose power. . . ."

During a cleanse, when you feel like resting, take a
few minutes for a nap or meditation and pause to appreciate
the good that is being accomplished by the release of toxins.
Buckminster Fuller knew the value of the semiconscious
resting place between sleep and wakefulness. He developed
a method to capitalize on this most creative, insightful time.
His technique was to lean back in a high-back leather chair
so that his head was supported, place a couple of small balls
in his hand, and drift off as deeply and quickly as he could.
If he fell asleep, the muscles of his hand would relax and the
balls would fall and wake him instantly. As he heard the
noise of the balls hitting the floor, he awakened rejuvenated
and refreshed. Even closing your eyes, leaning back, and
taking a deep breath can give you an instantaneous recharge. Or better yet, stand up and stretch your face and
arms to the sky while rooting your feet into the Earth.

Frequently during the day, humans build up tension throughout their bodies. Muscle tension creates acidic metabolic waste products that further irritate the musculoskeletal system and the subconscious. Taking a few minutes to focus on relaxing that tension will enable you to sustain a higher energy level and feel better during your busy schedule. Try one of the following exercises next time you need a break.

Neck Roll/Shoulder Lifts

Sitting or standing, close your eyes and inhale deeply, filling your lungs and belly. Slowly exhale, dropping your head forward, chin to your chest. Inhale deeply again while slowly rotating your head to the left, ear to your shoulder, and breathe normally as you feel the stretch. Lift your chin slightly to rotate and stretch your head up, then slightly to the back if comfortable (keep breathing!), then roll your head over to the right shoulder without dropping your head backward. Make three slow circles to the left, breathing deeply all the while, then circle to the right three times. Remember to breathe!

Next, scrunch up both shoulders toward your ears, squeezing tight and concentrating all of your neck and shoulder tension; hold for a moment, then release your shoulders down. For maximum benefit, inhale deeply as you draw your shoulders up and squeeze; exhale completely — even noisily, if you want — as you release. Repeat approximately eight times.

Progressive Relaxation

If you can lie down for a few moments, or at least rest back with your head supported, try this one. Beginning with your feet and working up your body, tighten each area of your body, one part at a time, to its maximum degree of tension. Then let it go, either quickly and completely or slowly and gently, and wait a few seconds, enjoying the new sense of relaxation in that part of you. When you have tensed and relaxed each part of your body, tense and release your entire body and then rest in this state of tension-free bliss. You can pop a progressive relaxation tape into your cassette player to guide you through this process (see appendix 1 for ordering information).

Self-Approval

As I mentioned at the beginning of this chapter, your mind can be your greatest enemy, but also your strongest ally. We have a tendency to judge ourselves harshly and to drive ourselves to some distant ideal of perfection. This behavior creates a state of mind that says we never have enough and we are never good enough.

Stop a moment and feel how your body feels when you judge yourself. It doesn't feel good, does it? Now change that feeling to one of love, approval, and appreciation for the great person you are and for the wonderful things you do. Now how do you feel? You can take this positive feeling and direct it inward to restore and revitalize your health.

Sleep

When doing your cleansing program, you may need more sleep than at other times, especially during the first few days. Often I think that the psychological component of changing habit patterns and wrestling with your mind to accomplish this wears you out, but there are also good physiological reasons for needing more rest. Your body is busy eliminating toxins and waste that have been housed in your tissues for years. Resting allows your body to concentrate its energy on this cleansing process. To get a more restful night's sleep, try stretching the progressive relaxation technique described a few paragraphs earlier or the Inner Smile process described below before you get into bed.

LET THE INNER SMILE TRANSFORM YOU

From the ancient Taoist system of healing comes a simple practice called The Inner Smile. Smiling into your abdomen and into the rest of your body is one of the quickest and most economical ways to change your mood and your physical state.

Master Mantak Chia, director of the Universal Tao Center and Tao Garden and author of numerous books on healing and meditation practices, teaches the Inner Smile, a powerful tool for self-healing. Chia says, "Smiling to yourself is like basking in love; you become your own best friend!"

Take a few moments and try this simple meditation. It will guide you through a process of smiling into every cell of your body for rejuvenation and healing. (To order an audiocassette of this relaxing and healing meditation, see appendix 1.)

Wear comfortable clothing, and sit relaxed in a chair. You can also try this practice lying down, but you risk falling asleep from becoming so relaxed. Place your hands comfortably in your lap, your right palm on top of your left. Breathe easily from your abdomen and gently close your eyes. Imagine that you are with someone you love or in a beautiful place in which you feel peace and joy. Picture yourself smiling, lift up the corners of your mouth, and feel the smiling energy in your eyes, too. Allow this energy to begin to soak into your body through a point between your eyebrows or on the top of your head. (One of my students felt best imagining the energy flowing into his heart.) Feel the energy flow like a waterfall down your face, into your eyes, relaxing your jaw and face muscles. Everywhere the smile touches, you feel more relaxed and rejuvenated, more alive.

Let the smiling energy flow into your throat and neck, moving into and filling your heart. As your heart fills with the loving smile, thank your heart for working day and night to pump your blood, carry nutrients, and sweep away waste from every tissue, organ, gland, and cell. Smile into your heart until your heart smiles back at you. Next, let the smile spread out to both sides, into your lungs. Thank your lungs for supplying life-giving air to all the parts of your body. Let the smile fill your entire lungs, all the way up to and above your collarbones. Feel the smile gently flowing down your body like a warm and soothing waterfall, then bring it into your liver, kidneys, spleen, intestines, bladder, genitals, spine, muscles, tendons, ligaments, bones, nerves, lymphatic system, skin, fatty tissue, hair, nails—every cell. Smile into all of these areas until they smile back at you, and thank them for the tireless work they do to keep you alive and thriving. Enjoy the relaxation, tingling, and excitement that you feel throughout your body from being touched by the smile—your smile.

When you have filled yourself with your smile and absorbed all of the goodness from it, bring your attention to your navel. Imagine that you have a ball or a treasure chest directly behind your belly button. Allow the excess bounty of the smiling energy to collect inside that place.

End your Inner Smile session by imagining a spiral at your navel, first in one direction then the other, to lock away the bounty until you need it. If you start to feel run down during the day, bring your attention to that magic place and draw out some smiling treasure to restore your health and vitality.

You can take half an hour or just a few seconds to enjoy the benefits of the Inner Smile. Why don't you pause for just a moment and lift up the corners of your mouth with a smile and feel your eyes smiling too? Let that smile wash over your entire body, mind, and soul. Inhale and feel it being absorbed into all of your tissues. It's as simple as that. Isn't that a great way to bring you back to what is important? Do you feel more centered and ready to go forth with your life? Can you imagine stringing a few of those moments together in your day? How would it feel if you were able to stay in this smiling state for an hour, or for a day?

For those of you who are more skeptical, just the thought of reaching inside your belly for treasure to enliven your day might give you a chuckle and help to change your state for the better. There is scientific, measurable evidence that your physiological state changes because of a shift in your hormones when you smile. When you smile, not only does "the whole world smile with you," but "smiling hormones" are produced and released into your bloodstream. Hormones have powerful effects on your mood, thoughts, and behavior. Why not make them "happy hormones"?

When people are depressed, their immune system is compromised. I am reminded of a Peanuts cartoon in which Charlie Brown is talking to a friend. He has his head hung low, slumped onto his chest, and he says, "This is my depressed stance. When you're depressed, it makes a lot of difference how you stand. . . . The worst thing you can do is straightening up and holding your head high because then you'll start to feel better. . . . If you're going to get any joy out of being depressed, you've got to stand like this."

Smiling and standing up straight, with your head held high, allows you to lighten up and appreciate the good things in life instead of filling your cells with the toxic chemistry of negative thoughts and feelings.

CONCLUSION

Allopathic medicine works on a model of removing symptoms. If you have a headache, a fever, diarrhea, constipation, irregular heart beat, or high blood pressure, for instance, you are given a drug to stop the unpleasant manifestation of your internal disorder. If you have a growth, polyp, tumor, congested gallbladder, or damaged intestinal tract, it will be cut out without a thought as to why the problem has occurred. Instead, we should be asking questions: What is behind all of this dysfunction and disease? What is the fundamental reason that we lose our health and become sick?

As you have learned by reading this book, our environment plays a major role in the state of our health. Yet human beings have been in challenging or toxic situations since time immemorial, and some have the amazing ability to thrive as demonstrated by human achievement as described in the following stories.

We hear of mothers who lift automobiles off their children who are pinned underneath. Thomas Edison tried over two thousand experiments before his invention, the light bulb, worked. A young reporter asked him how it felt to fail so many times. He said, "I never failed once. I invented the light bulb. It just happened to be a two-thousand-step process." Beethoven progressively lost his hearing. He was completely deaf by the age of forty-six, yet his greatest works were written in his later years. Franklin Roosevelt was paralyzed by polio at the age of thirty-nine, yet he went on to become one of America's most loved and influential presidents.

Wilma Rudolf was the twentieth of twenty-two children. Her survival was questionable right from birth. At age four, she became paralyzed in her left leg after a bout with double pneumonia and scarlet fever. At nine years of age, she took off her brace and began to walk. At thirteen she decided to become a runner. For the next few years, she finished last in every race she entered. After she eventually won a race her career skyrocketed, culminating in her winning three Gold Medals at the Olympics.

In *Spontaneous Remission: An Annotated Bibliography* by Brendan O'Regan and Caryle Hirshberg, you can read about a psychologist with rectal cancer. His doctor recommended immediate surgery. He refused any medical treatment, but sought the guidance of a therapist who taught meditation. Three hours of meditation every day reversed the debilitating complications of the rectal cancer, allowing him to return to his profession and continue with his favorite sport, hang gliding.

Do you remember the biblical story of Job? Job was a rich man with a loving wife and family until pestilence came upon him. He lost all of his material possessions. His neighbors and even his family turned their backs on him. He lost his health and still he would not despair; he continued to have faith. Finally all was restored.

There is within each of us a life force beyond what we eat, drink, or take in the form of pills that ensures our survival and gives us the ability to thrive. It cannot be measured by any of our scientific instruments, and doctors are not able to predict who will be able to mobilize this force to heal. What is evident is that those of us who feel loved and who focus on our health have a better-than-average chance.

I hope that you are now inspired and motivated to begin an internal cleansing program. Hundreds of thousands of people with a myriad of ailments have performed one form of cleansing or another over the millennia, and have benefited from the resulting renewed health and vitality. My own results and those of my clients and patients motivated me to share this information with you.

Never before have we been so in need of this knowledge. With the plethora of dangers that threaten our world today, it is easy to overlook the ills festering inside ourselves. As one woman said after completing her two-month cleansing program, "It's almost scary to see what you carry around inside, and it's a terrific feeling to know you got rid of that awful stuff." Other patients have said, "I began to feel better all over, and I have acquired a new energy," and, "It's like being reborn. I can't remember the last time I felt so good and had so much energy." There are many more testimonials from patients and clients who have had their lives changed by internal cleansing. From arthritis to allergies, whatever your problem, a good, safe cleansing program is sure to help. Your age or state of health doesn't matter. You can begin today to rebuild your own health.

Please do not postpone enjoying life until some future day when you are totally detoxified and have everything you could want in your life. Take action steps to minimize or eliminate the causes of your distress. Look for joy, peace, and happiness now. It may not be available in the outside world, but it is available every moment inside of you.

When the world deals you lemons, make lemonade. *Carpe diem!*

You may reach Dr. Linda Berry at:

1301 Solano Avenue
Albany, CA 94706
510-526-6657

or

712 D Street, Suite L
San Rafael, CA 94901
415-456-1300

or

Visit her Web site at
www.drlindaberry.com

Dr. Berry is available for workshops, talks,
consulting, and individualized treatment
programs (in person or by phone).

Appendix 1: Resources and Products

General

Anatomy

If you desire further information on the location of your body parts, *The Anatomy Coloring Book* (Addison Wesley, 1993) by Wynn Kopit and Laurance M. Ellson is a great resource for learning more about your body. The material is presented in a simple, easy-to-understand format.

Introduction

Health Coach Information

To support your cleansing process, my recommendation is to seek out a Health Coach in your area. The collective purpose of Health Coach is to teach, inspire, and support people to improve the quality of their health by improving the quality of their living. Health Coaches are committed to enriching lives through education and natural therapies.

If you would like to learn more about the internal workings of the human body, I would refer you to some of the educational tools available within the Health Coach System. *Functional Dietetics* is the most comprehensive guide today on dietary habits with respect to health. Learn the fundamentals of nutrition, what constitutes a complete diet, what role digestion plays and how you can improve yours, what detoxification is, how you can change your health, what role food allergies or intolerances play and how you can identify them, the role your doctor can play with respect to your nutrition program, and perhaps most important, what foods enhance healing and what foods lead to disease.

You may reach Health Coach by calling 888-888-8565 or on the Web at www.healthcoach.com to locate a trained Health Coach professional in your area or to obtain educational materials.

Chapter 1: Four Kinds of Stress

Biochemical Stress

Contact the Environmental Working Group, www.ewg.org, a non-profit environmental research organization based in Washington, D.C. They are a public interest watchdog. If you are chemically sensitive and would like to contact others like yourself try this e-mail support group: Cyndi@immune web.org; Web site: www.immuneweb.org.

In Dallas, Texas, Dr. William Rea supervises cleansing programs using nutritional supplements, exercise, and sauna therapy at The Environmental Health Center. You may contact Dr. Rea's office by calling 214-368-4132, Monday through Friday, 9 to 5; Saturday, 9 to 11.

Mental/Emotional Stress

Health Coach offers some excellent tools in this arena of healing. *The Mind-Body Connection* is a four-part video series and study guide that can help you approach your health and healing with renewed awareness and vitality by learning the action steps that leaders in the field of mind/body medicine are using to improve their clients' health. You may access these materials from a Health Coach in your area. To find one call 888-888-8565.

The language you use can serve to support your well-being, but too often it undermines your dreams and your self-confidence. *Power Talking,* an eight-part audio series by George Walther, helps you transform your culturally entrenched, negative, and powerless language into a dynamic vocabulary that will fuel your success. These materials are available from www.georgewalther.com, 425-255-2900.

CHAPTER 2: HOW THE BODY PROCESSES FOOD AND TOXINS

Thyroid Blood Tests

For more in-depth information on thyroid blood tests, contact:

> The Broda O. Barnes, M.D., Research Foundation, Inc.
> P. O. Box 110098, Trumbull, CT 06611
> 203-261-2101
> www.brodabarnes.org

If you suspect a low-functioning thyroid, the Foundation can help you locate a doctor in your area who has been trained in recognizing and treating this hormone imbalance. Their doctors also work with other endocrine or hormonal problems besides thyroid challenges to help you to find a balance in your entire hormonal system.

There are many types of thyroid therapy. Metagenics makes a product called Energenics, which supports thyroid function. Please call Metagenics at 800-692-9400 to find a health-care provider in your area who carries this product.

Antibiotics and Ear Infections

Learn why antibiotics may not be the best course of therapy for chronic ear infections, and discover other options, by reading *Childhood Ear Infections* (Group West, 1990) by Dr. Michael Schmidt.

CHAPTER 3: NATURAL ELEMENTS OF A CLEAN BOWEL

Essential Fatty Acids

You can get flaxseed meal with a nutty rich flavor from Omega Nutrition in your health food store or by calling 800-661-3529, and if you need inspiration on how to use it purchase a cookbook called *Flax for Life! 101 Delicious Recipes and Tips Featuring Fabulous Flax Oil* by Jade Beutler.

Dr. Donald Rudin and Clara Felix have recently published *Omega 3 Oils to Improve Mental Health, Fight Degenerative Diseases and Extend Your Life* (Garden City Park, NY: Avery Publishing Group, 1996) — an update of their book *The Omega 3 Phenomenon* (NY: Rawson, 1987). It is a very valuable resource for the way fats affect your health and well-being.

You can research the processing of oils in more depth in *The Facts About Fats* by John Finnegan (Berkeley, CA: Elysian Arts Books, 1993), who made an exhaustive study of oil-processing plants, visited researchers, read numerous volumes, and reviewed hundreds of original research articles to bring you this valuable information.

If you can't get your children to eat fresh flaxseed oil, try Essential Balance Junior from Omega Nutrition. And for yourself, use plain flax oil for the first 3 months to get your omega-3 balance up, then switch to Essential Balance Oil made in a 1:1 omega-6 to omega-3 balance. Or if you like that south of the border taste try their Flax Oil with Garlic and Chile. (To order or for more information, call Omega Nutrition at 800-661-3529.)

If your children still won't comply, perhaps you can encourage them to take a capsule of DHA in a supplement called Neuromins, a vegetarian source of EFAs from Martek. You may also contact Martek for a brochure about the value of EFAs in your infant's development at 800-662-6339. For more information on EFAs, see appendix 2.

High-quality oils are available from few sources; contact Omega Nutrition (800-661-3529) and Barlean's (800-445-3529) for your best options.

CHAPTER 5: HOUSEHOLD AND OTHER PERSONAL TOXINS

Water Filtration

To filter chlorine from your shower water, the Pure Water Store in Greenbrae, California, sells filters to fit shower-heads for less than $50. To purify the water you use for drinking and cooking, they have national associates who can sell and service combination charcoal carbon/reverse osmosis filters to fit under your sink. You may reach them by calling 800-776-7654.

If you are chemically sensitive and would like to contact others like yourself try this e-mail support group: cyndi@immuneweb.org; Web site: www.immuneweb.org.

Organic personal care products and medical supplies such as respirators and respiratory supplies are available from www.Tikvah.com.

Nirvana Safe Haven sells air and water filters, and organic beds and bedding on the Web at www.nontoxic.com.

Minimizing Pesticides

McKenzie Rock Flour is derived from basalt and andesite rock deposits of the Cascade Mountains of Oregon. I interviewed the owner of Remineralization Products, Inc., Lee Poindexter, and am satisfied that this is a sustainable product that does no harm to the environment or wildlife. You can order rock flour from Dan Weber, an independent distributor of McKenzie Rock Flour, by calling 800-339-0141.

Other staple ingredients in the pesticide-free war against insects include garlic, vegetable soap, chile peppers, Epsom salts, and mulch.

Gardens Alive! is a company dedicated to increasing fruit and vegetable yields and increasing the beauty of lawns and flowers by using natural compounds complementary to the Earth. The intent is to allow nature to find its balance, but when it needs help, to gently intervene. The first line of defense is to feed your plants to keep them healthy and strong enough to deter pests and environmental stressors like frost. The second line of defense is natural pest predators such as ladybugs, green lacewings, and birds. Gardens Alive! sells lacewings and lady beetles, but not birds. The third stage is to create barriers or traps to cut down on pest damage. These run the gamut from electronic flea catchers to pheromone lures to attract pests that would otherwise destroy fruit crops, and super-light barrier cloths that allow sunlight in to the plants while keeping crop-destroying insects out. As a last resort, they recommend using pest-killing plant or mineral compounds that break down quickly and are not harmful to people or the planet. You may contact Gardens Alive! to request a product catalog by phone: 513-354-1482; fax: 513-354-1484; or mail: 5100 Schenley Place, Lawrenceburg, IL 47025. And you may reach them on the Web at www.gardens-alive.com.

To find out more about the Bio-Integral Resource Center (BIRC), call 510-524-2567 or view their Web site at www.birc.org.

Rodale's Organic Gardening Publications are another excellent source of natural pest control options. For more information, visit their Web site at www.rodalepress.com.

Yale University offers yet another option: Change the nature of the typical suburban landscape. Their recommendations come in the form of a book called *Redesigning the American Lawn: A Search for Environmental Harmony* (New Haven, CT, and London: Yale University Press, 1963) by F. Herbert Bormann, Diana Balmori, and Gordon T. Gebalbe.

Mercury Amalgam Fillings

One way of telling if your body is saturated with mercury is to have a hair analysis done by a reputable lab such as Doctor's Data in Texas (800-323-2784). This test is not fail-safe, however. If you are a sensitive person, even test results "within normal limits" may be cause for mercury toxicity in your system.

Mercury Detox, a nutritional supplement that helps chelate mercury from your cells, is available from Integrative Therapeutics 800-869-9705.

I recommend three books on the subject of amalgam fillings: *Dental Mercury Detox* and *Dentistry Without Mercury* (Bio-Prove, 1995) by Sam Ziff and Michael F. Ziff, and *It's All in Your Head* (Group West, 1993) by Hal Huggins.

CHAPTER 7: DIETARY FIBER FOR GOOD HEALTH

Colon Care Formula is sold in health and natural food stores, and made by Yerba Prima (800-488-4339; Web site: www.yerba.com).

Nutri Flax is made by Omega Nutrition (800-661-3529; Web site: www.omeganutrition.com).

Meta Fiber is distributed by Metagenics (800-692-9400; Web site: www.metagenics.com).

CHAPTER 9: AN HERB AND FIBER CLEANSING PROGRAM

Women's Renew and Men's Rebuild Internal Cleansing Systems are available in health and natural food stores, or from Yerba Prima in Oregon (800-488-4339; Web site: www.yerba.com).

FOS Probiotic Growth Complex

Ultra Flora Plus is available in regular and dairy free forms for the dairy sensitive person. In order to find someone in your area who carries these products, call Metagenics at 800-692-9400.

CHAPTER 10: THERAPEUTIC FOOD POWDERS FOR CLEANSING

The Ultra Clear line of products is distributed by Metagenics (800-692-9400).

CHAPTER 11: CLEANSING THE LIVER AND THE LYMPH SYSTEM

Liver Cleansing

Dr. Elson Haas has written about liver-cleansing in his book, *Staying Healthy with the Seasons*. You may utilize his book for further guidance.

The liver cleansing properties of milk thistle, also called Silymarin, are available in tincture, tablet, and capsule forms in health food stores, or direct from Metagenics at 800-692-9400. The new, more bioavailable form of milk thistle seed extract is available as Milk Thistle Extra Strength from Yerba Prima at 800-488-4339; Web site: www.yerba.com).

Detoxification Factors (Integrative Therapeutics) can be found in doctor's offices or call customer service at 800-869-9705.

Cleansing the Lymph

Adopted by Applied Kinesiology, information on Chapman's Reflexes can be found in the book *Touch for Health* (DeVorss and Company, 1996) by Dr. John Thie.

For more information, see Charles Owen's compilation "An Endocrine Interpretation of Chapman's Reflexes" from the American Academy of Osteopathy 1992.

CHAPTER 13: DIET AND RECIPES

Nutrition

Contact Health Coach/NutriScan at 888-888-8565 or at www.healthcoach.com. To work directly with Dr. Berry use access code "health2090" after you enter the site for patients.

Great Plains Bentonite is sold in health and natural food stores, and made by Yerba Prima (800-488-4339; Web site: www.yerba.com).

Cleansing Diet

Dr. Jeffrey Bland has written a book called *The 20 Day Rejuvenation Diet Program* (New Canaan, CT: Keats, 1997) with Sara Benum, M.A. In this helpful book, Dr. Bland offers an easy-to-follow holistic prescription for turning around the "walking wounded" syndrome, wherein you don't feel well but the doctors say nothing is wrong and/or the prescribed medical interventions are not helpful for turning your symptoms around. Bland outlines a diet program that uses specific foods to counteract metabolic poisons and simultaneously provides the correct balance of nutrients needed by your body. Foods high in beta-carotene and vitamin C are central to the 20 Day Rejuvenation regime. Dr. Bland supplies a shopping list and daily menus (complete with recipes) for readers to follow. He also suggests a regular exercise routine, as physical activity helps eliminate toxins. Packed with personal stories, case studies, and self-evaluation quizzes, *The 20 Day Rejuvenation Diet Program* is for anyone who's trying to recapture physical and psychological zest. Based on clinical experience with thousands of patients who experienced significant health improvement, this consumer-oriented program uses specific rejuvenation foods and phytonutrients in a diet plan carefully designed to prevent problems of accelerated aging and to enhance your energy and vitality.

CHAPTER 14: SUPPLEMENTS TO SUPPORT CLEANSING

Daily Nourishing Tea

You can purchase this delicious combination of gently cleansing and nutritive herbs by calling Apothecary Tinctura at 800-220-5838.

Probiotics

To order Herbal Guard, contact Yerba Prima at 800-488-4339 or visit their Web site at www.yerba.com.

For Metagenics products, call 800-692-9400.

In Case of Oxidative Stress: Nutrients to Quench Free Radicals

If you have oxidative stress, what are some solutions? In doctors' offices you can purchase Oxygenics by Metagenics, a complete relay team of nutrients to quench free radicals. Many companies have developed antioxidant formulas. The best ones, like Oxygenics, will contain taurine, n-acetyl cysteine, glutathione, and alpha lipoic acid for special support of phase II detoxification in your liver.

Most of the phytonutrients named in chapter 11 are available in a product called Phyto Complete by Metagenics. Although it can't replace whole foods such as fruits, vegetables, nuts, seeds, grains, and legumes, Phyto Complete can offer a helping hand. If you don't always eat as well as you would like, this would be an excellent supplement for your nutritional support program. It comes in powdered or tiny pill form. If you are unable to find this valuable food in your area, call Metagenics (800-692-9400).

Chapter 15: Practices That Complement Cleansing

Behavioral Change Instruction

If you have a conflict between managing your career and managing your health, Stephen Covey's audio tape or book *Principle Centered Leadership* (New York: Simon and Schuster Trade, 1992) can help you to prioritize what is important to you. Order from your local bookseller or at www.amazon.com.

Anthony Robbins is a master at helping people change limiting behaviors and patterns. My synopsis of what Mr. Robbins teaches is stop complaining, take responsibility, and take action. If you need help in these areas contact his organization at 800-898-8669 or on the Web at www.tonyrobbins.com.

Exercise

Another great resource for health and vitality, including movement, is *The Power of Five: Hundreds of 5-Second to 5-Minute Scientific Shortcuts to Ignite Your Energy, Burn Fat, Stop Aging and Revitalize Your Love Life* (Rodale Press, Emmaus, PA: 1995) by Harold Bloomfield, M.D., and Robert Cooper, Ph.D. Their subtitle best describes what is offered in this useful guide.

For those who want more information on how to safely and effectively stretch to relieve tight muscles, look for *Stretching (20th Anniversary Edition)*, by Bob Anderson, Jean Anderson (Illustrator), Paperback, June 2000.

Deep Breathing

The Tao of Natural Breathing (Mountain Wind Publishing, 1997) by Dennis Lewis, emphasizes breathing with the whole body. Here's a quote from an article by Dennis about his new book: "I began to understand that superficial breathing ensures a superficial experience of ourselves, whereas natural breathing opens us to our own inner spaces and to the energies of the universe."

For more mind/body coaching and information, try the *Yoga Journal.* For more information visit their Web site at www.yogajournal.com or call 800-600-YOGA.

Rest and Relaxation

You might try *Progressive Relaxation and Autogenic Training* (relaxation CD) by Carolyn McManus, PT, MA, MS (www.anxietypanic.com/106.html). Or in book form try

Progressive Relaxation and Breathing by Matthew McKay (New Harbinger Publications, 1986).

   If you would like to contact The Healing Tao Center for information, a catalog of books, a schedule of classes, or a referral to an instructor in your area, please call 888-444-7426. You may also log onto www.universaltao.com or www.healingtaousa.com.

The Inner Smile

"The Inner Smile" is available on a two-sided audio cassette from www.drlindaberry.com. Side one guides you through a process of bringing healing energy into your organs, digestive system, and spine, then into every system and cell in your body. Side two has two shorter healing exercises. "Smile into Your Distress" assists you in dissolving the hold that stressful situations have on you. The second one, "Smile into Ecstasy," increases the joy in your mind, body, and heart.

APPENDIX 2: INFANT CARE

Infant Nutrition

Sources of the products found in the baby formulas in appendix 2 are as follows:

> Thorne: 800-228-1966 or 208-263-1337; Web site: www.thorne.com; e-mail: info@thorne.com
> Metagenics: 800-692-9400 or 949-366-0818; Web site: www.metagenics.com
> Scientific Botanicals (for the vitamin K drops) 206-527-5521 fax: 206-526-7948

The Thorne products and Source naturals DHA can be ordered through: Emerson Ecologics: 800-654-4432; Web site: www.emersonecologics.com

Flax Oil can be purchased at most health food stores or ordered direct from Barleans: 800-445-3529; fax: 800-551-9879; or Omega Nutrition: 800-661-3529

To order Neuromins, call Martek at 800-662-6339.

Metagenics (800-692-9400) has an excellent, well-tolerated (even in the first trimester of pregnancy when some women are experiencing nausea) prenatal supplement available through doctors' offices.

APPENDIX 2: INFANT CARE

Even commercial baby's milk is "rich" in toxic materials. If you choose not to breast-feed your infant or need to supplement with formula, please heed the following recommendations.

Stay away from premixed formula in cans. There is a high likelihood that the cans are coated inside with a plastic resin. You don't want to expose your little one to that hormone-altering material.

Read the ingredients. When I was doing some research in my local drugstore, I was surprised to find that sugar was included in some of the formulas. Corn syrup was the first ingredient in one of the non-dairy formulas. All of them contained vegetable oil (see appendix 3). What I have said in this book about commercial vegetable oils— the way they have been produced and the damaging effects they can have on a body—should raise a red flag. There are no "good" substitutes for a mother's milk. However, sometimes, such as in the case of adoption, there is no other alternative. In cases such as these consider the following recommendations.

HEALTHY BABY FORMULAS

A fortified Medipro formula may be your baby's best option if you are unable to breast-feed your infant. Dr. Timothy Birdsall and Dr. Alan Miller, naturopathic physicians and advisers to Thorne Research Inc. (a nutritional products company), analyzed mother's milk and devised a formula whose nutritional makeup is comparable to breast milk. The base is the Medipro Infant Formula produced by Thorne. The following easy-to-follow recipe provides you with an alternative to commercially available hypoallergenic infant formulas at about half the cost. This formula is made up of two parts: a dry powder mixture and a liquid oily mixture. These two parts are mixed together with maple syrup and water to make the final formula used for bottle-feeding. The texture is smooth enough to use in supplemental nursing systems.

Dry Powder Mixture

1 jar (18 oz.) Medipro
45 capsules Calcium CitraMate (160 mg of elemental calcium per capsule; 7,200 mg total)
5 capsules taurine (500 mg/capsule; 2,500 mg total)
9 capsules L-carnitine (350 mg/capsule; 2;970 mg total)
1 teaspoon "lite" salt (sodium potassium chloride)

Mix all powdered ingredients thoroughly and pour into original Medipro jar.

Liquid Oily Mixture

1 quart flaxseed oil
2 drops vitamin K_1 (2 mg/drop; 4 mg total)
2 capsules vitamin E (500 IU of d-alpha tocopherol* per capsule; 1,000 IU total)
30 capsules vitamin D_3 (400 IU/capsule; 12,000 IU total)

Mix all liquid ingredients thoroughly and store in an opaque container in the refrigerator.

Note: Use dl-alpha tocopherol (synthetic vitamin E) for a more hypoallergenic formula.

To make 1 quart of infant formula, combine 2 heaping table-spoons of the dry powder mixture with 7 teaspoons of the liquid oily mixture. Add 5 tablespoons of pure grade B maple syrup (sweetener and carbohydrate source) and enough water to make 1 quart total volume. (Grade B maple syrup has more nutrients than grade A.)

My friend and colleague, Ritamarie Loscalzo, M.S., D.C., CCN, DACBN, has used Medipro formula success-fully with her two adopted sons. To improve the essential fatty acid content, she also adds 1 capsule (100 mg) of Source Naturals DHA (docosahexaenoic acid) and ½ to 1 teaspoon of Metagenics Ultra Bifidus Dairy Free powder. Formula-fed babies need Ultra Bifidus to establish normal intestinal flora ("good bugs"); breast-fed babies get this bac-teria from their mothers in breast milk.

Dr. Loscalzo has found that preparing this 3- to 4-week supply (depending on how much the baby eats) takes only 30 minutes. And once a day, it takes only a couple of minutes to mix up 1 quart of infant formula in a blender. After the dry and liquid parts are mixed with the maple syrup and water, the formula must be refrigerated.

The Medipro Infant Formula is a predigested milk-based whey protein with some vitamins and minerals. Thorne com-pletely hydrolyzes the milk protein to a molecular weight of less than 10, which makes this product virtually non-allergenic. (Normal milk protein has a molecular weight greater than 100.)

Dr. Loscalzo's sons were fed this Medipro formula from birth. They were gradually transitioned to the Nut/Seed

Milk Formula (recipe below) beginning at 6 to 8 months, when they were comfortably able to handle solid foods. By one year, they no longer received the Medipro formula, but the formula is easy to make and may be continued until up to age 2 years of age.

When the baby is about 6 to 8 months old, you may begin to substitute puréed dates (½ cup soaked in ½ cup of hot water until soft) for the maple syrup in the Medipro formula because of the whole-food value they provide.

All-organic ingredients are best for your baby. Infants are especially sensitive to pesticide and herbicide residues in commercial products.

Dr. Loscalzo's Nut/Seed Milk Baby Formula

1. Soak 1 cup of raw nuts, seeds, or a combination in purified water for 6 hours or overnight. (Dr. Loscalzo most often uses a combination of almonds and sunflower seeds. Walnuts and pumpkin seeds are good too, because of their high fatty acid content. Small seeds such as sesame don't blend as well as larger seeds.)

2. Soak ½ to ⅔ cup of dates, pits removed, in 1 cup of hot pure (or purified) water.

3. Rinse the nuts and/or seeds well in pure water.

4. Blend the nuts and/or seeds in 2 cups of pure water or fresh vegetable juice. (Vegetable juice greatly enhances the nutritional value of the formula but also changes the flavor. Start to give juice when infants are 6 to 9 months old, when they haven't developed distinct preferences yet and usually

like the taste. Use at least half carrot and other mild vegetables, such as cucumber and celery. You may even add a little bit of beet. Add an apple to the mixture when using strong-tasting vegetables to sweeten the juice a bit.)

5. Strain the mixture into a large bowl or a 1-quart measuring cup. Squeeze out as much liquid as possible, then return the pulp to the blender.

6. Add 1½ cups of pure water to the pulp, and blend.

7. Strain the mixture well, and return the pulp to the blender.

8. Add the water that the dates have been soaking in, and blend once again.

9. Strain the mixture well, and discard the pulp. (If there is still a lot of pulp remaining, return it to the blender with ½ cup of pure water and blend. Strain, and discard the pulp.)

10. Return the liquid to the blender and add the following:

> Soaked dates
> 1 to 2 dropperfuls of Metagenics Mycelized Children's Multivitamins
> 1 tsp. Metagenics Ultra Bifidus DF
> ⅛ to ¼ tsp. Thorne Calcium Magnesium Citrate powder (between 65 and 130 mg of calcium)
> 1 teaspoon Metagenics Zinc Drink
> ¼ tsp. of the contents of a Thorne Iron Citrate capsule (5 mg of iron)
> 5 capsules of Source Naturals DHA (500 mg of DHA)

11. Do not strain the juice after adding the supplements.

For a quicker version of Dr. Loscalzo's Nut/Seed Milk Baby Formula, eliminate steps 5 through 9 and instead, do the following step after step 4, then jump to step 10: Blend well. If mixture seems too thick, add extra water or juice to desired consistency. You can also strain the mixture to thin it and discard the pulp or use in another recipe.

If you have any questions, you may contact Dr. Loscalzo by email at DrRLoscalzo@austin.rr.com.

MORE OPTIONS FOR BABY FORMULA

If you are not concerned about the allergenic quality of whole milk, you have another option. Whole Foods supermarkets distribute an organic whole-milk baby formula. They represent the formula as having a nutrient profile identical to infant formulas but advise use for 1 year and up, once the child is eating solid food. (For ordering information for the aforementioned products, see appendix 1).

Carnation Good Start is the best of the *commercial options* for baby formula if breast-feeding is not an option. The sweetener is lactose, which is healthier than sugar or corn syrup unless the infant is lactose-intolerant. The protein comes from lactalbumin (a milk protein) that has been partially digested to make it less allergenic.

EFAS FOR BABIES' DEVELOPING BRAINS AND BODIES

To compensate for nutrition lacking in a formula, you can supplement feedings with some of the products mentioned in this book, especially flaxseed oil or DHA and bifidobacteria (at any age). With respect to the flaxseed oil, for 11 to 22 pounds of body weight, ⅓ teaspoon per day will do; you can feed your baby the fresh oil with a spoon or rub twice as much directly onto his or her skin. For 22 to 33 pounds of body weight, use ⅔ teaspoon; and above 33 pounds, use 1 teaspoon for each 33 pounds of body weight.

It may be safer and more effective to use the DHA product Neuromins produced by Martek (see appendix 1). Neuromins is an omega-3 essential fatty acid concentrate made from an ocean algae source. The best source of this important nutrient is a baby's mother. Unfortunately, because of changes in our diet, mothers now have only half the level of DHA they had 50 years ago. Essential fatty acids from flaxseed oil or DHA are needed for the optimal development of a baby's brain and eyes. Sixty percent of the brain is made up of fats, and DHA is the most abundant fat in the brain. Other body tissues and fluids that have a high concentration of DHA are the heart, liver, and semen. DHA also supports immune system function and the health of baby's skin. The World Health Organization recommends approximately 10 milligrams of DHA for every pound of body weight. This means a 10-pound baby would need a minimum of approximately 100 milligrams of this essential fatty acid.

There is scientific evidence that the DHA a pregnant mother takes crosses the placenta to nourish her baby's brain. Martek recommends that pregnant and lactating moms take 200 mg of Neuromins each day because they are feeding half their supply to the fetus or newborn. Neuromins are available in health food stores. You may also be able to purchase it through a doctor's office that is on the cutting edge of nutritional science. If you are unable to locate DHA, you may find it on the Web at www.drlindaberry.com.

In 60 countries around the world, including Israel and countries in Southeast Asia and South America, all infant formulas are supplemented with DHA. Why don't American babies get the same consideration? Martek has applied for the Generally Accepted as Safe (GRAS) status for DHA in infant formula so that in the future, DHA may be included in infant formulas. Henry "Pete" Linsert, CEO for Martek, expects that infant formula supplemented with DHA will be available in the United States in 2001. In Asian countries, fish oil, which is high in EPA (another omega-3 oil) as well as DHA, is included in their infant formulas. EPA retards growth, however, possibly by interfering with arachidonic acid, another important fat for the developing brain. DHA is safer for babies.

International studies going back 20 to 30 years show a dose-dependent response with respect to the DHA content in baby's pre- and postnatal diets. That means that the greater the dose of DHA, the greater the response in terms of visual acuity and mental development as measured by the Mental Development Index of pre-term infants.[1,2] Normal-term infants who were breast-fed for up to 8 months showed linear improvement in long-term development up to 9 years of age.[3]

The omega-3 oil status of the developing fetus depends on that of its mother. However, pregnancy is associated with decreased omega-3 status. Often, mothers don't have enough time between births to replenish omega-3 body stores. There are lower omega-3 levels in second, third, and fourth siblings. This results in first-born children doing better than their younger siblings on several developmental, behavioral, and intelligence tests.[4,5] The kinds of fats a mother eats has a profound influence on her developing fetus. Americans eat too many altered or trans fats, including hydrogenated, partially hydrogenated, and fractionated fats (noted on nutrition labels). Cardiovascular risk may be programmed during early development.[6] We know that trans fats increase cardiovascular risk as reflected by the plasma lipoprotein profile.[7]

A deficiency of omega-3 fats has been reported in the blood plasma of people with cystic fibrosis (CF). The fat imbalance was observed in organs damaged by CF, including lung, pancreas, and intestines. Oral administration of DHA to mice corrected this fat imbalance and reversed the damage to these tissues.[8] Changing the levels of omega-3 fats may affect the lungs' response to infection. Animals placed on DHA-deficient diets exhibited inflammation of their bronchial tubes (a form of bronchitis) and were unable to mount a normal immune system response to fight the infection.[9] Based on this research, clinical trials have begun at Rush Presbyterian to study the effects of supplementation with 1-gram doses of DHA on people with CF.

For more information about the positive health benefits of DHA supplementation for your child, contact Dr. William Sears, a pediatrician and author of many books on children's health, on the Web at www.DHADoc.com or Martek Biosciences Corporation, www.martekbio.com, 410-740-0081.

HEALTHY "BUGS" FOR YOUR BABY

Mother's milk is high in bifidobacteria, which demonstrates immune-supportive effects. (Read more about this and about nourishing probiotic formulas in chapter 11.) I recommend using probiotics only from Metagenics because of the care they take to ensure the purity and efficacy of their products. In doctor's offices, you can find bifidobacteria in a product called Ultra Bifidus. If your baby is sensitive to dairy products, you can purchase this product in a dairy-free version. Use ¼ teaspoon three times per day. If you are breast-feeding but your newborn needs an extra immune-system boost, you can make the powder into a paste with a little water and rub it onto your nipple for your baby to eat while he or she nurses. If you are using formula, mix it right into the bottle. The bifidobacteria must be refrigerated.

If your infant is not dairy-sensitive, you can also add Probioplex Intensive Care from Metagenics. This product is especially good for relieving diarrhea. Give your child half the adult dose: ½ tablespoon, one to two times per day. These products are not harmful in any way as long as you follow the mentioned precaution with dairy-sensitive in-fants. They will only add to your baby's health and well-being. Probioplex Intensive Care has the advantage of not needing refrigeration.

Don't worry about mixing up these recommendations. The labels tell you what to do, except that the dose for your infant is half of the adult dose. Remember: Although your baby does not weigh half of what an adult weighs, if you were breast-feeding, your baby would be getting these nu-trients in large quantities from breast milk. Proportionately, babies need a larger amount than adults because of their de-veloping digestive and immune systems. Acidophilus supple-ments will be of no use to your baby until the baby is 2½ to 3 years old. (To purchase Metagenics products, call 800-692-9400 to find a health-care practitioner who carries them in your area.)

Appendix 3: Essential Fatty Acids and Omega-3 Supplements

I have taken flaxseed oil for a long time, but until reading *The Omega-3 Phenomenon* and speaking to Fred Rohe and reading his book *Eat Fat: Your Life Depends on It*, I was taking too little for my weight. When I increased my dosage the changes I enjoyed were amazing. The dry skin on the back of my arms, which manifested as little rough spots by the hair follicles, has become softer, smoother, and more silky to the touch. I notice that I remember phone numbers better when I am calling someone; I don't have to look at the number twice to complete dialing. My muscles feel stronger, and I am more stable on my feet; I haven't been leaning against the chiropractic table so much when working on patients. And I am waking up earlier with a clear head, feeling rested. The proper dose of flaxseed oil has already added considerable value and zest to my life.

Health Benefits of EFAs

In their book, *The Omega-3 Phenomenon*, Dr. Donald Rudin and Clara Felix outline the benefits of omega-3 fatty acid supplements:

1. skin improvements such as softer, smoother, firmer, flawless skin with improved tone and color, reduced sun sensitivity, and some fading of age spots on the hands
2. shinier, thicker, fuller hair
3. vitality, a zest for life, and increased stamina that lasts for long periods of time
4. smoother muscle action leading to greater agility
5. elimination of binging and the addictive need for food
6. reduction or elimination of food allergies
7. improved resistance to some diseases
8. improved functioning of the digestive tract, avoiding gas, constipation, and other disorders
9. stronger cardiovascular system
10. increased fat metabolism
11. clearer thinking
12. increased resistance to cold weather
13. increased physical comfort
14. improved quality of life

Felix and Rudin say that if you include omega-3 fatty acid supplements in your daily diet, you can expect benefits in as little as 2 hours; in some cases, improvement may continue for 1 or 2 years before leveling off.

Felix and Rudin did not include information in their list about the anti-carcinogenic effects of taking a flaxseed oil supplement. More recent research shows that omega-3 fatty acids kill human cancer cells in tissue cultures without destroying the normal cells in the same cultures. Breast, lung, and prostate cancer cells were studied. Omega-3 fatty acids lower high blood pressure and triglyceride levels. They decrease the probability of a blood clot blocking an artery in the brain (causing a stroke), in the heart (causing a heart attack), in the lungs (causing a pulmonary embolism), or in other organs (causing peripheral vascular disease such as gangrene).

Moreover, a study by J. J. F. Belch entitled "Effects of Altering Dietary Essential Fatty Acids on Requirements for Non-Steroidal Anti-Inflammatory Drugs in Patients with Rheumatoid Arthritis" (*Annals of Rheumatic Diseases,* 1988) showed that by using a combination of the omega-3 and omega-6 fatty acids, rheumatoid arthritics were able to completely discontinue or decrease their nonsteroidal anti-inflammatory drugs (NSAIDs), such as aspirin, Tylenol, ibuprofen, and Motrin. This is a very good thing because NSAIDs inhibit your liver's ability to process poisons from food, water, air, perfumes, colognes, body lotions, potions, and creams that you come into contact with or that you put on your skin on a regular basis. According to a November 1, 1995, article in *Family Practice News,* "One-fifth of all drug reactions reported to the Food and Drug Administration involved NSAIDs."

In addition to all of these benefits, Martek, the company responsible for championing the addition of omega-3 oils to infant formula (see appendix 2 for more information), performed studies in which they were able to raise red blood cell DHA from 2 to 8 percent with a dosage of 25 to 200 mg per day. Red blood cell DHA is a measure of the EFA content in your body. So the study showed that by taking DHA supplements, you do indeed raise the levels of these life-improving oils in your body.

THE IMPORTANCE OF BALANCED EFAS

Much of the information about fatty acids shared here comes from discussions with Fred Rohe and from reading his book, *Eat Fat: Your Life Depends on It*. Rohe discusses the optimal balance between omega-6 and omega-3 EFAs. Experts vary in their opinion of what is the best ratio. The ratio in your body tissue is 4:1, except in the brain and sex glands, where it is 1:1. The Standard American Diet (SAD) is grossly imbalanced, with a ratio of between 10:1 and 20:1.

Your body has different needs at different times, so it is impossible to always be perfect about the ratio of EFAs that you consume. Rohe recommends eating a variety of oils and taking an EFA supplement with a good average ratio of 2.5 omega-6 to 1 omega-3 EFAs to ensure an adequate supply of EFAs for most people most of the time. Children need EFAs, too. To encourage brain development, use a 1:1 ratio until puberty.

- For a 1:1 ratio, mix 3 parts fresh flaxseed oil with 2 parts fresh sunflower oil.
- For a 2:1 ratio, mix 1 part fresh flaxseed oil with 2 parts fresh sunflower oil.
- For a 3:1 ratio, mix 1 part fresh flaxseed oil with 3 parts fresh sunflower oil.

Remember, though, that you are probably starting with an imbalanced fatty acid status. If a core sample of your fat could be taken, it would tell you just what type of fats you have been eating. Because most fats and oils in the marketplace are trans fats, which are destroyed by processing or hydrogenation, you are probably severely deficient in EFAs—especially omega-3. A period of supplementation with fresh flaxseed oil exclusively, which is in a 1:3 omega-6 to omega-3 ratio, while eliminating trans fats from your diet, will help to improve your body fat constitution and your health. Continue with the flaxseed oil alone for 3 to 6 months. If you continue to eat a significant amount of omega-6 oils by eating out a lot or consuming quantities of sunflower or sesame seeds or any other oil than flaxseed oil, you may need to continue with fresh flaxseed oil with its 1:3 ratio over the long term.

BUY HIGH-QUALITY OILS

In order to ensure that you are eating only high-quality oils, look for oils that:

- are processed below 118°F
- are processed excluding light and air
- are processed without toxic solvents
- are bottled in opaque containers
- have air displaced by inert gas

Fats are altered not only by the processes mentioned above, but also by the normal processing that all but a few brands undergo. Oils, even those sold in health food stores, are expeller-pressed, with presses the size of railroad cars subjecting them to temperatures of up to 180°F, and filtration through phosphates and caustic sodas. Bleach deodorizing further raises the temperature to 520°F. If the oil is produced by a large commercial company, it will also be run through a solvent extraction using hexane—a volatile liquid paraffin hydrocarbon found in petroleum—to increase the oil yield and their profits. Expeller-pressed "natural brands" undergo the same process, minus the hexane treatment. They may

even call this oil "cold-pressed" because there are no regulations about what "cold-pressed" means. The end product—
the oil you buy at the market—has minimal nutritional value
and little similarity to real food. Nutrients are either altered
or removed and, to amplify this transgression against human
health and well-being, it contains poisonous trans fatty acids,
free radicals, and other toxic substances. Periodic cleansing,
supplemental nutrients, and high-quality oils help to prevent
the damage of this now-unavoidable material—commercially
processed vegetable oil.

EFAs are sensitive to damage from heat and light,
which is why it is important to process them below 118°F
and to store them in opaque containers. Opaque plastic is
the material of choice for those companies that produce
fresh oils. Most oil is sold in clear or tinted glass bottles,
which exposes them to enough light to change their chemical composition, producing toxic, cancer-causing substances. The metal tins in which much olive oil is stored also
damage the oil. The solder that holds their seams together is
probably made from tin and lead—not optimal for contact
with your food.

APPENDIX 4: TESTS AND SELF-EXAMS

TEST YOUR ESSENTIAL AND METABOLIC FATTY ACIDS

Fatty acids were once thought to be no more than stored calories. However, current research is finding out that essential fatty acids (EFAs) are some of the most important nutrients in the human diet, critical for the walls of your cells, for their function, and for hormone signaling. The number of diseases affected by EFA therapy is huge, including inflammatory disorders, cardiovascular disease, hormonal disorders, auto-immune disorders, and many cases of senile neurologic degeneration.

Changes in the modern diet are largely responsible for the increasing incidence of EFA imbalances and deficiencies. The ratio of omega-6 to omega-3 fats has changed drastically as a result of the widespread use of vegetable oils (mostly omega-6 vegetable fats) in cooking, and the processing of oils to alter omega-3 fats to improve shelf life and eliminate their strong taste. In fact, historical estimates place the ratio of omega-6 to omega-3 oils at nearly 1:1 for prehistoric humans, but by the beginning of the twentieth century, this ratio had increased to about 4:1. Estimates for Americans in the early 1990s placed the ratio in the range of 20:1 to 25:1.[1] The sharp rise is due to increased vegetable oil consumption: from 2 pounds per year in 1909 to 25 pounds per year in 1985.[2] The ideal dietary ratio should probably be in the range of 1:1 for the brain, eyes, testes, and heart, and 4:1

for muscles; a minimum of 1 percent of our diet should come from omega-3 oils.[3]

In a study of 847 patients aged 50 to 70, 322 patients had at least one EFA outside the normal range. Of those 322 patients, 57 percent of them had at least two abnormal values. General trends observed included an increase in abnormal values with age, as well as increases in heart disease and cancer.[4]

The cutting-edge technology that allows laboratories to measure EFAs in membranes has become available only within the past couple of years. Today, however, Great Smokies' state-of-the-art Essential and Metabolic Fatty Acid Analysis offers physicians a precise assessment of 30 individual fatty acids and five of the important ratios (such as the ones influencing chronic inflammatory conditions), as well as percent distributions of fat families, including the omega-3 and omega-6 fatty acids.

To test for red blood cell fatty acids, a fasting whole blood sample is required. To find a doctor in your area who performs this test, contact Great Smokies Diagnostic Laboratory in Asheville, North Carolina, at 800-522-4762.

TEST YOUR pH LEVEL

The pH of each portion of the gastrointestinal (GI) tract is critical for the activation of the various digestive juices. The mouth and esophagus—the tube running between your mouth and stomach—optimally maintain a neutral pH of 7.0 to 7.2. You can check the pH of your own mouth with litmus paper (ordering instructions follow). You can also use litmus paper to perform the following simple experiment, which will indicate whether you have a "health reserve."

1. Put a small piece of litmus paper in your mouth and determine the pH by comparing the color against the color chart on the litmus paper container.
2. Cut off a slice of fresh lemon and suck out all of the juice.
3. Swish the juice around in your mouth, then swallow it.
4. Wait one minute (60 seconds).
5. Retest your pH by placing another piece of litmus paper in your mouth.
6. Compare your pH to the pH you noted before sucking the lemon.

Has your pH increased, stayed the same, or dropped relative to your original reading? Your findings can be likened to a financial portfolio. If your pH stayed the same, it's like living from check to check and having only enough money to cover your expenses. If your pH increases above the optimal range, you have "savings" to increase your current well-being and security in times of stress. On the other hand, if your pH dropped below optimal, you are running up your "debts" and moving toward "bankruptcy" unless you begin to make some significant changes.

You can get litmus paper from your local pharmacy or order it direct from:

Micro Essential Laboratory, Inc.
4224 Avenue H
Brooklyn, NY 11210
Phone: 718-388-3618
Fax: 718-692-4491

TEST YOUR LEVEL OF DIGESTIVE ACIDS

The next portion of the GI tract, the stomach, must be acidic (have a very low pH) to stimulate the more alkaline secretions of the small intestine. If your stomach acids are weak, your body has no impetus to produce strong alkaline (or basic) enzymes.

To determine whether your digestive secretions are low, observe whether and when you get gas after a meal. Gas soon after eating is a sign that your stomach secretions are low. If you get gas within an hour or two after eating, then your small intestine's digestion is probably deficient. A Health Coach can help you assess the state of your digestion by taking a history, completing a thorough physical examination, and reviewing questionnaires that you have filled out prior to your visit. Or else schedule a visit with a gastroenterologist.

Laboratory tests are available but are invasive and costly. The Heidelberg test for adequate stomach secretions is performed by placing a capsule down your throat and esophagus into your stomach. The capsule acts as a transmitter, and a receiver in the room where the test is conducted picks up information from the capsule and measures your stomach acidity or lack thereof. An osteopath friend who conducts the test says that the procedure can sometimes take 2 hours. At least one of my colleagues believes that this test is inaccurate because having an object stuck down your throat and into your stomach puts you into an alarm state that shuts down your digestive juices.

TEST YOUR LIVER FUNCTION

If you would like to find out how your liver is functioning, contact Great Smokies Diagnostic Laboratory for a licensed health-care professional in your area who works with these tests (800-522-4762). One of the nice things about Great Smokies' stool test is that they check to see which pharmaceutical drugs and natural herbal substances destroy the harmful microorganisms found in your stool sample. Many of the findings in their Comprehensive Digestive Stool Analysis measure your level of protective substances against cancer of the breast, prostate, and colon compared with what would be found in a healthy person. Because these cancers are great killers in our population, it makes sense to find out where you stand if you want to live a healthy, vibrant life. If the profile doesn't look good, you can then get some good advice from a natural health-care professional or make necessary changes on your own, such as the ones recommended in this book, to restore your vibrant health.

TEST YOUR LARGE INTESTINE

The final portion of your intestines, the colon, may also be evaluated for a variety of markers that are indicative of health or disease through stool analysis. This valuable test is done by many progressive doctors, *and* you have to collect the stool sample and send it off to the lab in a timely manner so that the results will be accurate. I recommend Great Smokies Diagnostic Laboratory for this test. After carefully analyzing 6 tons of samples last year, they have established themselves as the leaders in the field of stool analysis and functional body assessments. You may reach them by calling 800-522-4762 and asking for customer service. They will be happy to put you in touch with a licensed health-care professional in your area who uses this technology.

Two major tests evaluate the status of your lower GI tract: the Comprehensive Digestive Stool Analysis and the Intestinal Permeability Test. The Comprehensive Digestive Stool Analysis evaluates digestion, absorption, intestinal function, and the microbial fauna. GI disorders have a major impact on health. One recent study found that in nearly 70 percent of American households, at least one person had experienced one or more GI symptom during a 3-month period.[5]

The Intestinal Permeability Test determines underlying problems linked to GI function. It directly measures how well two non-metabolized sugars permeate the intestinal mucosa. One sugar, mannitol, is a small molecular weight molecule that should pass easily through your intestinal lining. The other, lactulose, is a large molecule. It passes through your gut into your urine if you have a leaky gut. To perform the test, the patient mixes premeasured amounts of lactulose and mannitol and drinks the substance, then collects a urine sample 6 hours later. The test measures the amount of lactulose and mannitol recovered in the urine sample.

Malabsorption and leaky gut have been linked to inflammatory bowel disease, inflammatory joint disease, food allergy, coeliac disease, use of non-steroidal anti-inflammatory drugs (NSAIDs), and more.[6-11]

Other tests performed by Great Smokies Diagnostic Laboratory useful in combination with those listed here are the Parasitology Profile and the Food Allergy Profile.

TEST YOUR LEVEL OF OXIDATIVE STRESS

Oxidative Stress Questionnaire

Point Scale

    0 = None or Never
    1 = Slight or Rarely
    2 = Mild or Occasionally
    3 = Moderate or Frequently
    4 = Severe or Almost Always

Answer each of the following questions relative to your symptoms or history over the past month. Once you've completed the questionnaire, ask a Health Coach or seek a health-care practitioner who can help you interpret the results.

1. ___ Do you have symptoms that are aggravated by air pollution?
2. ___ Are you sensitive to smoke, perfume, or other chemical odors?
3. ___ Do you have ongoing problems with fatigue?
4. ___ Do suffer from joint pain or deep muscle pain?
5. ___ Do you have a significant environmental exposure to pollutants (at work or at home)?
6. ___ Rate your use of tobacco products.
7. ___ Rate your exposure to second-hand smoke.
8. ___ Rate your consumption of alcoholic beverages.
9. ___ Rate your unprotected exposure to sunlight or ultraviolet light.
10. ___ Rate your level of exercise.

11. ___ What is your exposure to prescription drugs, over-the-counter medications, and/or recreational drugs?
12. ___ Rate your daily stress level.
13. ___ Rate your intake of fried foods, margarine, or high-fat foods.
14. ___ How often do you seek medical care or advice for your health concerns?

Add up the numbers to arrive at a total.
___ Total
Are you currently taking antioxidant supplements?
___ Yes ___ No

Reprinted by permission of HealthComm International, Inc.

In addition to the Oxidative Stress Questionnaire, objective laboratory tests can be performed to evaluate whether you are at risk for damage to your heart, lungs, GI tract, or nervous system from free radicals. Ask your health-care practitioner for details. You also can call Great Smokies Diagnostic Laboratory at 800-522-4762 for information about how the amount of oxidative stress in your body can be measured using blood and urine tests.

NOTES

CHAPTER 1

1. Angelillo IF, Villari P, Bull "Residential EMFs and childhood leukaemia: a meta-analysis." *World Health Organization* 1999; 77(11):906–15.
2. Dockerty JD, et al. "Electromagnetic field exposures and childhood cancers in New Zealand." *Cancer Causes Control*, May 1998.
3. Meinert R, Michaelis J. "Meta-analysis of studies on the association between electromagnetic fields and childhood cancer." *Radiation Environmental Biophysics*, Feb 1996; 35(1).
4. Miller MA, et al. "Variation in cancer risk estimates for exposure to powerline frequency Electromagnetic fields: a meta-analysis comparing EMF measurement methods." *Risk Analysis*, April 1995; 15(2):281–87.

CHAPTER 2

1. Smith MD, Gibson RA, Brooks PM. "Abnormal bowel permeability in anklylosing spondylitis and rheumatoid arthritis." *Journal of Rheumatology*, April 1985; 12(2):299–305.
2. Stefansson, et al. *Medical Intelligence;* 312(4).
3. Leirisalo-Repo M, Repo H. "Gut and Spondyloarthropathies." *Rheum Disease Clin North Am*, Feb 1992;18(1):23–25.
4. Inman RD. "Arthritis and enteritis—an interface of protean manifestations." *Journal of Rheumatology*. June 1987;14(3):406–10.

CHAPTER 3

1. Burkitt DP. "Related disease—related cause?" *Lancet*. Dec 1969; (7632):1229–31.
2. Siguel E. *Essential Fatty Acids in Health and Disease: Using the Essential Fatty Acids w3 and w6 to Improve Your Health , Lower Your Cholesterol and Prevent Cardiovascular Disease*. Nutrek Press, 1995
3. Erasmus U. *Fats That Heal, Fats that Kill: The Complete Guide to Fats, Oils, Cholesterol and Human Health*. Alive Books, 1999.
4. Finnegan J. *The Facts About Fat: A Consumers Guide to Good Oils*. Celestial Arts, 1993.
5. *Ibid*.

CHAPTER 4

1. Gunderson EL, FDA Total Diet Survey, April 1982–April 1986. "Dietary intakes of pesticides, selected elements and other chemicals." Food and Drug Administration, Division of Contaminants Chemistry, Washington, DC 20204.

2. Crinion W. "Environmental medicine, part 1, the human burden of environmental toxins and their common health effects." *Alternative Medicine Review*, 5(1): 20052–63.

3. Washington AP, 6/12/00 reported by Lauran Neergaard, AP Medical Writer

4. Ibid.

5. Chaudron LH, Jefferson JW. "Mood stabilizers during breastfeeding: a review." *J Clin Psychiatry*, Feb 2000; 61(2);79–90

CHAPTER 5

1. National Academy of Sciences Jan 19, 2000 press release. "Study Finds Strong Evidence that Exposure to Some Indoor Substances Can Lead to or Worsen Asthma." For more information call 800-624-6242 or 202-334-3313 or on the web contact news@nas.edu and ask for the brochure "Cleaning the Air: Asthma and Indoor Air Exposures."

2. Jacobson JS. Jacobson SW. "Evidence for PCBs as neurodevelopmental toxicants in humans." *Neurotoxicology*, 1987;18(2):415–24.

3. Ibid.

4. Davis JR, et al. "Family pesticide use and childhood brain cancer." *Arch Environ Contam Toxicol*, 1993; 24:87–92.

5. Leiss J, et al. "Home pesticide use and childhood cancer—A case control study." *Am J Public Health*, 1995; 85:249–252.

6. Crinion W. "Environmental Medicine, part 1: The human burden of environmental toxins and their common health effects." *Alt Med Review*, 2000; 5(1):52–63.

7. Claggett S. 2,4-D Information Packet. Northwest Coalition for Alternatives to Pesticides. 1990.

8. Wakefield AJ, et al. "Ileal-lymphoid-nodular hyperplasia, non-specific colitis, and pervasive developmental disorder in children." *Lancet* Feb 1998; 351(9103):637–41.

9. Crinion W. "Environmental medicine, part 1."

10. Haschek WM, et al. *Handbook of Toxicologic Pathology*. San Diego, CA. Academic Press. 1991.

CHAPTER 6

1. Dunnick JK, et al. "Assessment of the carcinogenic potential of chlorinated water: Experimental studies of chlorine, chloramine, and trihalomethanes." *J Natl Cancer Inst* 1993; 85(10):817–22.

2. Landi S, et al. "Induction of genetic damage in human lymphocytes and mutations in Salmonella by trihalomethanes: role of red blood cells and CSTTI-1 polymorphism." *Mutagenesis*, Sep 1999; 14(5):479–82.

3. Nieuwenhuijsen MJ, et al. "Chlorination disinfection by products in water and their association with adverse reproductive outcomes: a review." *Occup Environ Med*, Feb 2000; 57(2):73–85.

4. Cantor KP, et al. "Drinking water source and chlorination by products in Iowa. III. Risk of breast cancer." *Am J Epidemiol* 1999;150(6):552–60.

5. Sidhu KS, et al. "Need to revise the national drinking water regulation for copper." *Regul Toxicol Pharmacol.* Aug 1995; 22(1):95–100.

6. Dr. Joel Michalek, Air Force Health Study. Air Force Statement on Results from the 1997 Physical Examination of the Ranch Hand Study, Press Release Mr. 15, web site executive summary at www.brooks.af.mil/AFRL/HED /HEDB/AFHS/AFHS.shtml; for more informaion, contact Dr. Michalek at 210-536-2600.

7. Michalek J, et al. "Post service mortality of US Air Force veterans occupationally exposed to herbicides in Vietnam: 15 year follow-up." *Am J Epidemiol,* 1998; 148(8):786–92

8. Stephenson J. "IOM report links Agent Orange exposure to risk of birth defects in Vietnam vets' children." *JAMA,* 1996; 275(14):1066–7

9. Ziegler J. "Environmental 'Endocrine Disrupters' get a global look." *J of the Natl Cancer Inst,* 1997; 89(16):1184–1187.

10. Palmer JR, Rosenberg L. "Cigarette smoking and the risk of breast cancer." *Epidemiol Rev,* 1993; 15:145–156.

11. Wolff, MS, et al. "Blood levels of organochlorine residues and risk of breast cancer." *J Natl Cancer Inst,* 1993; 85:648–652.

12. Falck FY, et al. "Pesticides and polychlorinated biphenyl residues in human breast lipids and their relation to breast cancer." *Arch Environ Health,* 1992; 47:143–46.

13. Dewailly E, et al. "High organochlorine body burden in women with estrogen receptor positive breast cancer." *J Natl Cancer Inst,* 1994; 86:232–34.

14. Bertazzi PA, et al. "Cancer incidence in a population accidentally exposed to 2,3,7,8-tetrachlorodibenzo-para-dioxin." *Epidemiology,* 1993; 4:398–406.

15. Flesch-Janys D, et al. "Exposure to polychlorinated dibenzo-p-dioxins and –furans and breast cancer mortality in a cohort of female workers of a herbicide producing plant in Hamburg, Germany." *Proceedings of the 1993 Dioxin Conference, Vienna, 9 Sep 1993;* 381–84.

16. Manz A, et al. "Cancer mortality among workers in a chemical plant contaminated with dioxin." *Lancet,* 1991; 338:959–64.

17. Wolff MS, Weston A. "Breast Cancer risk and environmental exposures." *Environ Health Perspect NIH, Natl Inst of Environ Health Sci,* 1997; 105, suppl 4:891–96

CHAPTER 7

1. Dr. Christine Williams. Columbia University Children's Hospital, NY. "Dietary Fiber in Childhood: How much should be recommended." Vahouny Fiber Symposium, Vienna, VA, March 2000; 20–23.

2. Rose DP, et al. "Effects of diet supplementation with wheat bran on serum estrogen levels in the follicular and luteal phases of the menstrual cycle." *Nutrition* 1997; 13(6):535–9

3. Weisberger, et al. "Protective mechanisms of dietary fibers in nutritional carcinogenesis." *Basic Life Sci,* 1993; 61:45–63.

4. Rose DP, Connolly JM. "Dietary prevention of breast cancer." *Med Oncol Tumor Pharmacother,* 1990; 7(2-3):121–30.

5. Goldin BR, et al. "The effects of dietary fat and fiber on serum estrogen concentrations in premenopausal women under controlled dietary conditions." *Cancer*, 1994; 74(3 supl):1125–31.

6. Woods, et al. "Hormone levels during dietary changes in premenopausal African-American women." *J Natl Cancer Inst*, 1996; 88(19):1369.

CHAPTER 8

1. Sherdlow JL. "Nature's Rx." *National Geographic*, Apr 2000, 197(4): 101–2.

CHAPTER 9

1. Hoffmann D. *Holistic Herbal*. Element, 1996.

CHAPTER 10

1. Bland and Bralley. *Journal of Applied Nutrition*. 44(3 & 4), 1992.

2. Rigden S. "Entero-hepatic resuscitation program for CFIDS." *The CFIDS Chronicle*, 1995:46–9

3. Rigden S, MD, et al. "Evaluation of the effect of a modified enterohepatic resuscitation program in chronic fatigue syndrome patients." Functional Medicine Research Center, HealthComm International, Inc, Gig Harbor WA. Research Report 103, 1997.

4. Schlitz, RN, et al. "Tolerance, flavor acceptability, and general health observations of a newly developed children's medical food product called Ultracare for Kids." Functional Medicine Research Center, HealthComm International, Inc. Gig Harbor, WA, Research Report 100, 1997 January 17:1–16.

5. American Academy of Allergy and Immunology Committee on Adverse Reactions to Foods. "Adverse reactions to foods." NIH Publication No. 84-2442:43–85

6. Caffarelli C, et al. "Elimination diet and intestinal permeability in atopic eczema, a preliminary study." *Clin Exper Allergy*, 1993; 23:28–31.

7. Barau E, et al. "Modifications of intestinal permeability during food provocation procedures in pediatric irritable bowel syndrome." *J Pediatr Gastroenterology Nutrition*, 1990; 11:72–7.

8. Walker-Smith J. "Food sensitive enteropathy: Overview and update." *Acta Paediatrica Japonica*, 1994; 36:545–9.

9. Schlitz B. "Tolerance."

CHAPTER 13

1. Bland JS and Levin B. "Nutritional Therapy." *Encyclopedia of Alternative Medicine*. SP Creative Design, UK 1997.

2. Bidlack, WR. "Interrelationships of Food, Nutrition, Diet, and Health: The National Association of State Universities and Land Grant Colleges White Paper." *J Am Coll Nutr*. 1996:422–33.

3. American Dietetic Association Position Paper. "Position of the American Dietetic Association: Phytochemicals and functional foods." *J Am Diet Assoc.* 1995; 95:493–96.

4. Weisburger JH. "Approaches for chronic disease prevention based on current understanding of underlying mechanisms." *Am J Clin Nutr,* 2000;71 (6 Suppl):1710S–1714S.

5. Clement Ip, et al. "Trans fatty acids and cancer." *Nutrition Reviews* 1996; 54(5):138–45.

6. Bal DG, Foerster SB. "Dietary strategies for cancer prevention." *Cancer* 1993; 72(3 Suppl):1005–10.

7. Olga KA and Bullock JD. "Children with allergic rhinitis and/or bronchial asthma treated with elimination diet: a five year follow up." *Ann Allerg,* 1980; 44:273–78.

8. Philips DA. *Guidebook to nutritional factors in foods.* Woodbridge Press, Santa Barbara, CA, 1979.

9. Tucker KL. "Potassium, magnesium, and fruit and vegetable intake are associated with greater bone mineral density in elderly men and women." *Am J Clin Nutr,* 1999; 69(4):727–36.

10. "Fruits and veggies: bone boosters." *Health News,* 1999 May 10; 5(6):5.

11. Rao AV, Janezic SA. "The role of dietary phytosterols in colon carcinogenesis." *Nutr Cancer.* 1992; 18(1):43–52. Review.

12. Thomas HE Jr, et al. Cholesterol - phospholipid ratio in the production of coronary heart disease. The Framingham Study. *NEJM.* 1996 Mar 31;274(13):701-5.

13. Reynolds KD, et al. "Increasing the fruit and vegetable consumption of fourth graders: results from the High 5 project." *Prev Med,* 2000; 30(4):309–19.

14. Prestera T, et al. "Chemical and molecular regulation of enzymes that detoxify carcinogens." *Medical Sciences,* 1993; 90:2965–69.

15. Davis M, et al. "In vitro metabolism of cyanohydroxybutene: formation of a glutathione-s-transferase catalyzed product". *Research Communications in Chemical Pathology and Pharmacology,* 1993; 79(3):343–53.

16. Schiltz B, and Liska D. *The Rejuvenation Diet Study.* Functional Medicine Research Center. HealthComm International, Inc, Gig Harbor, WA. 1997 Jan 21 Research Report 101.

CHAPTER 14

1. Kaneda Y, et al. "Effects of berberine, a plant alkaloid, on the growth of anaerobic protozoa in axenic culture." *Tokai J Exp Clin Med,* 1990; 15(6):417–23.

2. Sheng WD, et al. "Treatment of chloroquine-resistant malaria using pyrimethamine in combination with berberine, tetracycline or cotrimoxazole." *East Afric Med J,* 1997; 74(5):283–84.

3. Hitokoto H, et al. "Inhibitory effects if condiments and herbal drugs on the growth and toxin production of toxigenic fungi." *Mycopathol,* 1979; 66(3):161–67.

4. Sohni YR, Et al. "The antiamoebic effect of a crude drug formulation of herbal extracts against Entamoeba histolytica in vitro and in vivo." *J Ethnopharmacol,* 1995; 45:43–52.

APPENDIX 2

1. Carlson SE, et al. "Longchain fatty acids and early visual and cognitive development of preterm infants." *Eur J Clin Nutr,* 1994; 48(suppl):27–30.
2. Carlson SE, Werkman SH. "A randomized trial of preterm infants fed docosahexaenoic acid until two months." *Lipids,* 1996; 31:85–90.
3. Lansing CL. "Neurologic differences between 9-year old children fed breast milk or formula-milk as babies." *Lancet;* 334(3):319–22.
4. Lucas A, et al. "Breast milk and subsequent intelligence quotient in children born preterm." *Lancet;* 339:261–4.
5. Gale CR., Martyn CN. "Breast feeding, dummy use and intelligence." *Lancet;* 347:1072–5.
6. Barker DJP. *Mothers, babies and disease in later life.* London: BMJ Books, 1994.
7. Mesnik RP, et al. "Dietary saturated and trans fatty acids and lipoprotein metabolism." *Ann Med,* 1994; 26:461–4.
8. Freedman S. "A membrane lipid imbalance plays a role in the phenotypic expression of cystic fibrosis in cftr-/-mice." *PNAS,* 1999; 96(24):13995–14000.
9. Harper TB, et al. *Am Rev Respir Dis* 126:540–7.

APPENDIX 4

1. Simopoulos AP. "Omega 3 fatty acids in health and disease and in growth and development." *Am J Clin Nutr,* 1991; 54(3):438–63.
2. Linder MC. "Nutrition and metabolism of fats." *Nutritional biochemistry and metabolism. 2nd ed.* Norwalk, CT:Appleton & Lange, 1991:51–83.
3. Innis SM. "Essential dietary lipids." *Present knowledge in Nutrition. 7th ed.* Washington, DC ILSI Press, 1996:58–66.
4. Shamberger RJ. "Erythrocyte Fatty Acid Studies in Patients." *J Advance Med,* 1997; 10(3):195–205.
5. Drossman D, et al. "US householder survey of functional GI disorders: prevalence, sociodermography and health impact." *Dig Dis Sci,* 1993; 38:1569–80.
6. Pironi L, et al. *Dig Dis Sci,* 1990; 35(5):582–8.
7. Bjarnason I. *J Rheumatol,* 1990; 17(20);38–41.
8. Rooney PJ, et al. *Clin Exp Rheumatol,*1990; 8(1):75–83.
9. Butkus SN, Mathan LK. *J Am Dietetic Assoc,* 1986; 86(5):601–8.
10. Pearson AD, et al. *Br Med J,* 1982; 285(6334):20–21.
11. Jenkins AP, et al. *Gut* 1991;32(1):66–69.

BIBLIOGRAPHY

Anand, Margot. *The Art of Everyday Ecstasy*. Broadway, 1998.

Ashley, Cynthia, and Sylvia Valazques. *Creative Reuse Extravaganza*. Oakland, CA: East Bay Depot for Creative Reuse, Inc., 1996.

Blair, Steven. *Living with Exercise*. Dallas, TX: American Health Publishing Company, 1991.

Beinfield, Harriet and Korngold, Ephrem. *Between Heaven and Earth: A Guide to Chinese Medicine*. Ballantine Books, 1992.

Benson, Herbert with Stark, Marg. Timeless Healing: *The Power and Biology of Belief*. Scribner, 1996.

Bland, Ph.D., Jeffrey. *The 20-Day Rejuvenation Diet Program*. New Canaan, CT: Keats Publishing, 1997.

Bloomfield, Harold and Cooper, Robert. *The Power of 5*. Rodale, 1995.

Borman, Herbert. F., Diana Balmori, and Gordon T. Geballe. *Redesigning the American Lawn*. New Haven and London: Yale University Press, 1993.

Colborn, Theo, Dianne Dumanoski, and John Peterson Myers. *Our Stolen Future*. New York: Dutton, 1997.

Covey, Steven. *First Things First*. New York: Simon and Schuster, 1994.

Erasmus, Udo. *Fats That Heal, Fats That Kill*. Blaine, WA: Alive Books, 1993.

Finnegan, John. *The Facts About Fats*. Berkeley, CA: Celestial Arts, 1993.

Galland, Leo. *The Four Pillars of Healing*. Random House, 1997.

Hirshberg, Caryle and Barasch, Marc Ian. *Remarkable Recovery*. Riverhead Books, 1995.

Jensen, Bernard. *Tissue Cleansing Through Bowel Management*. Escondido, CA: Bernard Jensen Enterprises, 1981.

Kapit, Wynn, and Lawrence M. Elson. *The Anatomy Coloring Book*. New York: Harper College Publishers, 1993.

Myss, Caroline. *Why People Don't Heal and How They Can*. Harmony Books, 1997.

O'Regan, Brendan, and Caryle Hirshberg. *Spontaneous Remission: An Annotated Bibliography*. Sausalito, CA: Institute of Noetic Sciences, 1995.

Owen, Charles. *An Endocrine Interpretation of Chapman's Reflexes*. Newark, Ohio: American Academy of Osteopathy, 1992.

Percival, D.C., N.D., Mark. *Infant Nutrition*. New Hamburg, Ontario: Health Coach Systems International, 1994.

Percival, D.C., N.D., Mark. *Functional Dietetics: The Core of Health Integration*. New Hamburg, Ontario: Health Coach Systems International, 1995.

Percival, D.C., N.D., Mark, and Cheri Percival. *Guilt Free Indulgence: A Cookbook with Conscience*. New Hamburg, Ontario: Health Coach Systems International, 1995.

Pert, Candace. *Molecules of Emotion: Why You Feel The Way You Feel*. Scribner, 1997.

Roth, Gabrielle. *Sweat Your Prayers: Movement as Spiritual Practice.* Tarcher Putnam, 1997.

Rudin, M.D., Donald O., and Clara Felix. *The Omega 3 Phenomenon.* New York: Rawson Associates, 1987.

Rudin, M.D., Donald O., and Clara Felix. *Omega 3 Oils to Improve Mental Health, Fight Degenerative Diseases, and Extend Your Life.* Garden City Park, NY: Avery Publishing, 1996.

Samuels, M.D., Mike, and Hal Zina Bennett. *Well Body, Well Earth.* San Francisco: Sierra Club Books, 1985.

Siguel, M.D., Edward. *Essential Fatty Acids in Health and Disease.* Boston, MA: Boston University Medical Center, 1994.

Thie, John. *Touch for Health.* Marina del Ray, CA: DeVorss and Company, 1995.

INDEX